TRUST SURRENDER RECEIVE

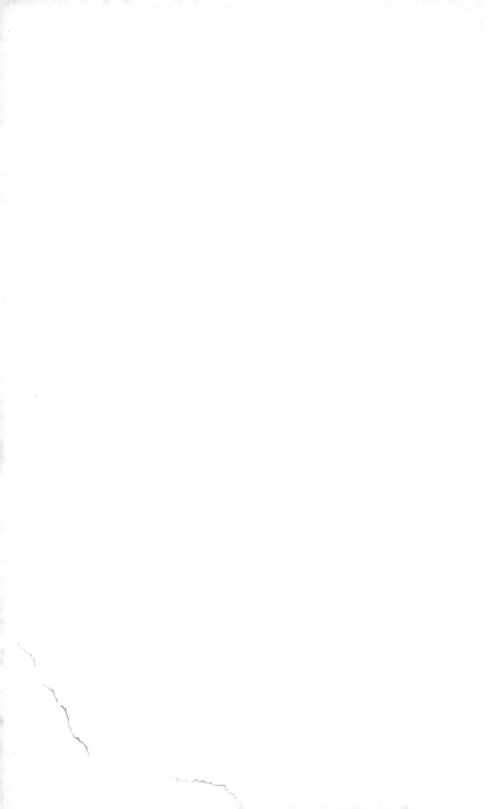

TRUST

SURRENDER

RECEIVE

How MDMA Can Release Us
From Trauma and PTSD

. . . . . .

ANNE OTHER

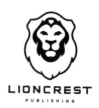

LIONCREST
PUBLISHING

TRUST SURRENDER RECEIVE
How MDMA Can Release Us From Trauma and PTSD

ISBN   978-1-61961-738-4 *Paperback*
        978-1-61961-739-1 *Ebook*

For Panda 1

This book is dedicated to those individuals who, through no fault of their own, have experienced trauma and lived their lives with its deleterious consequence, the ongoing and incessant symptoms of fear. From the seeming hopelessness of their situation, this exquisite medicine offers a universal hope of release from conditions we have come to accept as normative. Too many have passed without ever knowing of the healing potential of MDMA, and it is to bring this forbidden knowledge to the living population in great need that this book was written.

Contents

———

"All that was left was this anguished heart, eager to live, rebelling against the deadly order of the world that had been with him for forty years, and still struggling against the wall that separated him for the secret of all life, wanting to go further, to go beyond, and to discover, discover before dying, discover at last in order to be, just once to be, for a single second, but forever."

ALBERT CAMUS; THE FIRST MAN

Acknowledgements

This book would not exist without the steady and knowledgeable involvement of many individuals at Book in a Box and Lioncrest Publishing. From my nervous first conversation with Dan Bernitt outlining our thoughts about the book and his unequivocal acceptance of the project, through Kevin Murphy's plan of the book's shape and outline, to the many hours of focused work, week in and week out, with editor Sheila Trask, I have been supported with truth, constancy and good humour in a way that I could have only dreamed of.

From the broad overall view of the project to the smallest detail, their commitment never wavered in fulfilling my request to 'get this over the finish line'. In truth, without them and their designers, copy editors, and others involved the entire project would, at this very moment, be no more than many pages of scattered text.

Their utterly professional commitment to this project has never faltered even as it grew and grew beyond anyone's expectations, and their editorial insistence on the necessity of this or that element was always on point, tireless but never tiresome. This in spite of the fact that our working relationship was conducted without a single face-to-face meeting, over many months and across many, many miles.

What began for us as an obligation to share this work became an endeavor of truly overwhelming complexity, but once in their hands it was a calm, steady and seamless progression toward publication. With a deep bow to everyone involved, these few words are but a small token of my great respect, gratitude and appreciation.

ANNE OTHER

The Gift That Is MDMA

We are blessed to have in our possession a medicine that can release us from trauma and PTSD (Post-Traumatic Stress Disorder). We are also cursed by the fact that it is forbidden for our use, and in the considered opinion of many individuals, including those involved in the publication of this book, this prohibition is untenable.

In truth, MDMA (3,4-Methylenedioxymethamphetamine) may be one of the most extraordinarily useful and reliably effective psychological medicines ever to come into our hands, arguably on a par with physiological medicines such as penicillin, insulin, and morphine. It deserves, therefore, our utmost respect.

MDMA's psychic reach is boundless, its effects both gentle and powerful. Even though its mechanism-of-action has remained mysterious until now, the healing outcomes speak volumes. The testimonies in this book describe the benevolence of its action to release us from trauma and PTSD, and presents us with observational evidence of the truth of Dr. Ivor Browne's profound hypothesis, 'Psychological Trauma or Unexperienced Experience.'

With this lens, the capture and release of trauma becomes comprehensible, coherent, and explicit, expressed through the written experiences of over forty individuals who have exposed themselves to MDMA in therapeutic settings.

We invite you to share these experiences in their own words.

● ● ●

WHO WE ARE

"Nature abhors a vacuum."

ARISTOTLE

For six years following the collective trauma of September 11th, 2001, the individuals responsible for this book responded to requests from friends in need. Seeing their often-dire plight, we felt a sincere obligation to pay forward the benefits we had received from working with MDMA and were moved to honour their requests by sitting with them at this medicine work, as attendants.

Our decisions were not made lightly. However, knowing of the work's beneficial trajectory when administered by skillful means—and having, ourselves, experienced its lasting healing potential—the decision was essentially made for us. Individuals in severe, chronic, and treatment-resistant pain deserve to have access to every possible method to heal themselves. Regrettably, this is not the case. This remarkable medicine is currently prohibited and is characterised as having "a high potential for abuse" and "no currently accepted medical treatment use."

Prior to our own healing experiences with this *sui generis* medicine, we chose to do our due diligence by taking advantage of the wealth of public information to come to our own conclusions about the work. We knew from unbiased clinical research that toxicologists gave a clean bill of health to pure, medical grade MDMA, and our own experiences had borne this out. When approached by friends, who regarded us as having the skill-set necessary to administer the work, we responded with our hearts.

We come from all socio-economic groups and are as diverse as life allows; young and old, female and male, etc. This range allows clients to work with an attendant of their choosing, someone with whom they can identify and trust. Simply, our work is the work of human beings and their attentive presence.

ABOUT THE TESTIMONIES

"When the news is this good, you have to share it."

AN ATTENDANT

The testimonies in this book describe how each client approached the medicine work, their experience of the six-hour session itself, and descriptions of their outcomes. The task was to describe a little about who they were before the work, their experiences during the session itself, and some indication of how their lives may have been affected after the session. Each testimony was willingly offered by each client who chose either to write their own essay or to be interviewed.

A handful of testimonies are interviews conducted by a reporter who had, herself, experienced the work. The remainder are either self-penned essays or a spoken account transcribed and edited lightly for coherence, omitting no content. The attendant present at each session wrote a brief introductory and concluding paragraph to each edited testimony, which was then shown *in toto* to the client for approval. Revisions were honoured per the client's requests until they were satisfied that not only their words were authentic, but also that the attendant's comments were true and accurate. Each then chose a pseudonym by which they would remain unknown, thus completing their sign-off on their testimony.

In bringing these testimonies together for publication over the past few years, we have given considerable thought to how they might be categorised for the reader's convenience. This has proved a challenge. Arranging them according to the range of problems with which each client presented was one possible approach, but it is seldom the case that people come to this work with only one condition, and the variables prevented the possibility of categorisation. Similarly, with the medicine sessions and their outcomes, the range of experiences was simply too wide to have any value as categories. So, with the best will in the world, we have simply identified Men and Women with two sub-categories, Couples and Therapists.

Our motivation in publishing these testimonies is to introduce this medicine work to individuals who may have little or no idea of MDMA's healing potential. For us, this is work we respect as offering healing potential for trauma beyond anything currently available, and as such, deserves to be understood at face value.

This is not a book with a beginning, middle and end that needs to be read in a linear way from start to finish. The text will give some idea of the work, the bones, as well as the surrounding context, but the testimonies are the flesh and blood and sinew of this endeavour. Each of *them* has a beginning, middle and end, and it is by reading them in aggregate that readers will find the best opportunity to make sense of what this work is truly all about.

Having experienced the healing potential of MDMA themselves, these clients were adamant that good, true information about the medicine work needed to be shared, and their testimonies bearing witness were written to this end. This book has been prepared in the belief that it is only through first-person accounts that the elegance and sheer magnitude of MDMA's revelatory and healing potential can be credibly described. This book is a vehicle for these generous individuals to share their experiences in such a way that they may become comprehensible to a reader to whom the healing potential of this extraordinary work is unknown.

I had no experience with drugs at all.

Elly S.

The events Elly recounts in her testimony had already occurred, when we were introduced by her son. She had worked during the Schedule I prohibition in 1985 and seeing in person the outcome of her experiences with MDMA was inspirational and an important part of realising the possibilities for practical application of the healing potential of this medicine.

At ninety, Elly is more engaged with life than many people one-quarter her age, and her mature willingness to submit to the medicine in the first instance is evidence of the intensity of her life force. With little more than a trust in the process per Grof, she saw how anxiety had led to suicidal thoughts and shaped her life.

INTERVIEWER: I wanted to start with a bit of background information; where you grew up, how you became interested in singing and performing?

ELLY: I was born and brought up in Williamsburg (Brooklyn, New York City). It wasn't fashionable when I was a child. I always sang; my talent was sort of recognised by the family. My mother lost no opportunity to show it off. At the age of, I think, twelve, I got accepted into the High School of Music and Art; and in my junior high school, the music teacher took me home to meet her sister, Lillian Stronghan, a voice teacher who became my mentor. Ultimately, I considered her my real mother and still do.

She recognised she was dealing with a traumatised child and took me under her wing. I was raised in an abusive and loveless home. I do believe Lillie's interest in me and weekly visits to her home/ studio to sing and afterwards for coffee and talk, saved certainly my sanity and possibly my life. I say that because even with her help, and her being there for me, and the ultimate success I had, I was always plagued with depression and anxiety throughout my life. Thoughts of suicide were never far from my mind, but I think Lillie reaching me in my adolescence kept me from acting on it. Her teaching gave me purpose when the depression paralysed action.

It was when my career was tapering off, at the age of fifty-eight, that I found myself in a real crisis. That's when I decided it was about time to do something. I fortunately had a friend who had done psychedelic therapy in London in the late 1950s or early `60s. She knew Grof. She had become a psychologist; she shared her office with a psychiatrist friend. I got in touch with her, and we set up a time to do the work. My first session was on MDMA.

I: She believed MDMA would be the best medicine for you?

E: Yes, it is actually. I had never taken *any* drugs. I had no experience with drugs at all.

I: That's a big deal then.

E: It was quite big for me; I was really desperate. I had one request. I said, "I don't know where I'm going, but I want to hold Beethoven's hand. So, please play Beethoven for me, and I'll feel less frightened."

He played the wrong Beethoven. He played the 5th; I wanted the 7th, but it didn't matter. Suddenly, I'm catapulted into the kitchen of our apartment. I'm about five years old. (All our social life and family life was lived in the kitchen.) I got the most vivid picture of my mother coming through the door, exhausted, martyred, angry, and resentful. My father is standing with his back against the sink. She is angry; and obviously, they're angry with each other, and I'm standing in the background feeling this big. Children always feel they're the ones responsible, and they're unable to do anything about it. In that session, I realised my mother didn't love me. I never consciously knew that before. "My God, she didn't love me."

Well, that explains why I didn't like her. If a mother loves you, you damn well love her, and I felt very guilty then as a kid that I didn't. I never even admitted that to myself. I just wondered why I never had much feeling for her.

The *major* insight that came of this session was the realisation my entire life had been lived around the fulcrum of anxiety. What I now call and recognise as anxiety, I had oddly never named. I'm talking about a constant sense of unease, even a feeling of always wanting to jump out of my skin. It was such an everyday part of life for me, I assumed it was the way everyone lived. Of course, if that is so, you don't complain, because that is what it means to be alive. I never thought to question it, since I had never been without it. I assumed, so had everybody else.

From the very first session where I was taking MDMA, I realised the truth about my mother. I felt that it was about ten years of therapy in one session. It was amazing!

I went back the next day, crying. I said, "What am I supposed to do with all this? I'm fifty-eight years old. What am I supposed to do with this? What do you do at my age? I feel like I'm standing onstage and just dropped my drawers." And he said, "Look, I used to be a psychoanalyst, Freudian. I worked with people for years, and I was contemplating getting out of it; because some people I managed to help somewhat, but I didn't think talk therapy achieved that much." And he continued, "Then, I started working with Grof, and I began to see near miracles. My suggestion to you is go home with it, see what happens in the next two weeks." So, I did.

Before the session, I don't ever remember having a non-anxiety dream, ever.

Those dreams I remembered ranged from vaguely uncomfortable to very uncomfortable. After I left his office, I went home and lo and behold had the first dream I ever had that was not an anxiety dream. It was just factual. A couple of days later, I noticed there was no anxiety; it was gone. I suddenly felt comfortable in my skin. I was able to drop my shoulders. I was able to feel like a normal human being. Now, initially, the anxiety came back as high anxiety for specific things, but otherwise, it just went away; and after the second session, you know after a few weeks and after the next session, I had no anxiety at all really.

Because one of the major things this stuff does is rid you of a lot of fears.

Elly's indomitable spirit has brought her from a life of suicidal ideation and constant anxiety to a place where she can teach the singing in which she excels to students she loves. She is closely involved with her son and his family as a loving mother and grandmother. Her ongoing meditation practice enables her to maintain the balance she has achieved in this work and to be present for herself and others in ways that were unavailable to her as a younger woman.

What Elly found in this work was the eternal part of herself that is at peace, within which she was able to see the truth of her upbringing and to understand how this had impacted her entire life. Viva Elly!

Prologue

Astonishment is the only word to adequately describe what our clients express when they have experienced MDMA. If we are astonished in this work, it is because we, ourselves, are astonishing; our capacity for consciousness is boundless. The medicine gives us nothing except an extraordinary openness to ourselves, and every scrap and shard of the content that emerges is ours. Once seen, it is allowed to be released, resulting, (often for the first time in one's life), in a lifting of depression, anxiety, or fear. Clients are awed to find themselves, for the duration of the session and beyond, raised out of their personal darkness into a more wholesome, balanced, and optimistic state of mind.

Finding a medicine that can do that may seem unlikely, even impossible; but, in fact, we already have such a medicine, and we are not using it. The evidence supporting MDMA's use in the treatment of trauma is considerable, and trauma is implicated as the root cause of depression, anxiety, and fear. Yet, this pharmacological intervention is not currently sanctioned by the medical or legal communities.

OLD STORY, NEW DAY

"First, it is ridiculed. Second, it is violently opposed. Third, it is accepted as self-evident."

ARTHUR SCHOPENHAUER

Throughout history, new medical treatments have been met with suspicion. Consider the difficulties faced by London surgeons trying to perfect their surgical skills in the early 1800s, a time when they were both scorned by physicians and prohibited from cutting open human bodies by edicts from the Church of England. This prevented young, enthusiastic surgeons from gaining necessary experience and skill. Knowledge of anatomy was rudimentary, surgical conditions were appalling with no attention to hygiene, and medical progress relied upon people to do the work of examining the human body and seeing how the whole physical structure worked.

Surgeons-in-training needed cadavers on which to practice, so they had no choice but to go outside the law. The only way they could further their education was to engage a black market by hiring fringe members of society who were prepared to rob graves for them. Under cover of darkness, these individuals brought to the surgeons deceased human bodies.

Today, as head of the Church of England, the Archbishop of Canterbury is as likely to submit to the surgeon's knife as any other member of the public, and it is impossible to imagine how modern medicine would look if doctors had never had access to cadavers. How else could we have learned about human anatomy?

A similar prohibition exists in medicine today, but instead of the church barring the use of human bodies, government agencies outlaw research into, and use of, such medicines as MDMA. In the 1980s, therapists and clients alike lauded this medicine as an invaluable tool for understanding and ameliorating psychological problems, yet this view stood in direct opposition to the perception of legislators, law enforcement officials and social workers who dealt with fallout from the recreational use of MDMA-related substances at parties and raves. Some recreational users became ill or died, resulting in a backlash against this agent, despite the adulteration it had suffered en route to the recreational user. Ritalin, angel dust (PCP), caffeine, Adderall, and worse have been added to pure MDMA, compromising any sincere attempts to evaluate its true nature and confounding the ability of skilled practitioners, psychologists, and others to utilise it in their practices. Thus, for the past thirty years, we have been forbidden therapeutic access to a unique and potentially game-changing medicine.

It is the limits placed on MDMA that have led to an underground practice that, in an important respect, parallels the situation faced by would-be surgeons in the nineteenth century; practitioners must venture outside the law to practice their skills.

We are not healers. We have no training or skills that could heal anybody. What we do have, however, is the ability to be present for someone who is willing to expose her or himself to the medicine to *heal themselves.*

We do not act as therapists, suggesting an orthodox, interpersonal relationship with our clients, but fully embrace the descriptor "therapeutes." This Greek word is the root of our word therapist, but over time, its meaning has become compromised and obscured. The original meaning of the word therapeutes is 'an attendant at the healing process,' and that precisely describes our role. We only attend, minute by minute, to the healing process unfolding within the client.

Individuals who approach us have often been depressed, anxious, and fearful for years, and have tried most every other intervention to ease their suffering. One of the most salient characteristics of depression is the sufferer is convinced their hopelessly bleak worldview is the only one that exists. He or she cannot imagine a way out or have any means to consider the possibility of thinking in a wholesome, balanced, and optimistic way. All is darkness. However, after sessions with MDMA, these individuals may experience the light at the end of the tunnel for the very first time and, importantly, become able to carry this hope forward into their lives.

To provide a window into the way many of us came to this work, let's look briefly at how one of us came to act as an attendant:

"My involvement with MDMA began after many years of search-ing for relief from social anxiety and depression down traditional alleys. I did some cognitive behavioural work, went through talk therapy with a psychologist, and took a brief dip into the world of psychopharmacology, but none of these approaches solved my problems. Conventional psychiatry and psychology con-centrated on bringing the subconscious to the conscious mind to be known and cognitively examined; the premise seemed logical, but was not particularly effective. My brief foray into antidepressant medication simply left me with the feeling: 'Get me out of here.'

I realised I needed an experiential therapy to help me deal with chronic social anxiety and depression. The first was primal therapy, which encourages the participant to fully express whatever feelings come up—in my case, anger—in the safety of the treatment room. I also used breathwork, a breath-based active meditation process. This was very promising and effective.

Over time, I had become aware of the healing potential of MDMA. I approached a trusted friend and requested she sit with me for a session, and it was simply the most extraordinary experience of my life to that point. It is difficult to describe, but essentially, all the things I had been struggling with became absolutely manageable. MDMA puts you in another, special realm. Everything is the same on the outside, but inside, you inhabit another sensibility. One person has described it as discovering 'vistas of promise.' For me, it was, "Oh, I never knew I could feel this good. I never knew this existed. How come nobody ever told me about this?"

It is remarkable for a depressed and anxious person to try a new treatment and immediately experience such understandings. The word 'ecstasy,' which has been chosen to market street drugs related to MDMA, provides an apt description of the feeling clients report. MDMA also increases empathy, primarily toward ourselves, but also toward people who have been problematic in our lives. Finding oneself in this expanded state can recalibrate one's relationship with long-held traumas in a profound way. The trauma we have been unable to face gets reframed as something neutral, an event we can acknowledge and then move beyond. With MDMA guiding the ship, we can observe the trauma that is at the root of our troubles from a buffered distance. It is like watching a shark in a tank at the aquarium; the creature is clearly there in all its power and strength, but it is safely swimming behind sturdy glass walls, and we experience no fear. US President Roosevelt was right: "We have nothing to fear but fear itself."

In this way, under the benevolent influence of the medicine, we can access once-repressed traumatic material with remarkable clarity. We are no longer under threat, so we can look right at it, staying to examine the trauma without fear. Before MDMA, the fear level has been too high; with MDMA, examining the memory feels safe. The entire organism comes to understand the pain happened in the past, and what happened in 1992 is not still happening in 2017. In an action of release that conditions the client's astonishment, the body then lets go of its hold on what it captured, spontaneously releasing the trauma as decisively and completely as it captured it in the first place. The understanding of this biological mechanism comes from 'Unexperienced Experience.' Dr. Ivor Browne's hypothesis that will be addressed in Chapter Five.

The psyche, faced with a life-threatening event, cut us off from that traumatic memory, because it knew the memory was too much for us to handle. The event was simply too awful. After the event, unwittingly, we carry the ordeal around within us, possibly for decades and can only come to terms with it, and be released from it, when the psyche finally understands the threat has been removed, and that it is something from the past. The organism maintains hypervigilance, acting as if the threat is always present, until it is convinced otherwise.

Dr. Ivor Browne's revelatory hypothesis of 'Unexperienced Experience' lays bare the extraordinary mechanism of capture and release. His profoundly insightful hypothesis critically informs our work. When we expose ourselves to MDMA we open and observe the previously frozen event, (Browne calls it 'the frozen present'), not with trepidation but with a fierce fascination. Our ability to revisit the traumatic memory under the kind and patient medicine offers us new information that allows us to revisit the trauma itself from the buffered distance, and from this perspective, we can understand and be released from the trauma.

The reality of this experience will become clear throughout this book, through the testimonies of people who have experienced MDMA. In these pages, you will hear from people with a wide range of unique experiences with treatment-resistant trauma and its release through MDMA. One testimony, which follows next, comes from a person who went to a sleep clinic for insomnia, where he was told he had PTSD. He had never been to war, so the diagnosis seemed preposterous. On the other hand, he had lived in New York City at the beginning of the AIDS crisis and had seen friend after friend die of the disease. Over three sessions, he came to peace with losing those people from his life. He started the sessions by feeling as if all the young men he had lost were locked in a room. In the first, he opened the door and went into the room with them. By the sixth session, he went in and nobody was there. They were free. Not only are all his PTSD symptoms gone, he has no more insomnia.

People come to us to work with MDMA with different types of conditions, all of them products of trauma. A core trauma might produce depression in one person, anxiety in another, binge drinking or violence in yet another. Trauma is the root of our dysfunction. It is not a new idea; theories about the mental and emotional effects of repressed trauma go back to Sigmund Freud's early work in Paris with neurologist Jean-Martin Charcot. These founders of psychoanalysis understood trauma's central role in the formation of most neuroses. Today, we understand trauma sits at the base of a whole spectrum of disorders. Almost every condition listed in the *Diagnostic and Statistical Manual (DSM) of Mental Disorders* can be seen to stem from trauma.

If the theory of hidden traumas is not new to psychology, why have we not used agents like MDMA to release them before now? Is this medicine finally finding a foothold in trauma therapy despite the prohibitions against it? These are questions we'll address later; for now, consider the disconnected nature of our society, culture, and economy. The industrial revolution separated us from everything except efficiency; it cut us off from what it means to be truly human. Tools like MDMA can point us back to a more wholesome idea of ourselves and a more holistic way of functioning in the world.

In this regard, it is interesting to consider the word "educate." Our present system urges us to become educated and accumulate high school diplomas and undergraduate and graduate degrees by studying at colleges and universities. We are sent off to fill ourselves with whatever there is to be learned about our chosen field; we learn from existing knowledge and carry that forward into our careers. The modern meaning of the word "educate," however, has become radically detached from the word from which it is derived, essentially reversing its meaning. The original Latin word "educare" is compounded from two words, "e(x)" meaning "out of," and "duco," meaning to lead. Thus, the true meaning of the word educate is "to lead out of," specifically to lead out of each individual whatever it is that expresses that individual's unique abilities, talents, and personality.

In our view, the medicine work, as presented here, authentically expresses the true meaning of the word education.

A different kind of war, but a war nevertheless.

Carl B.

Carl is an actor whose career was blindsided by the AIDS crisis when he went to New York in the early 1980s. His testimony has directly inspired and given shape to this book, and we honour his courage to enter the work in the absence of little more than trust; in his referee, in his attendant, in the medicine, and in the process overall. Ditto his courage, unbidden, to share his experiences in order to make them explicit to others, and we cannot thank him enough for his generous act that has given birth to this collection of testimonials.

After we had worked three or four times, he came with a nine-page, single-spaced essay about what had happened to him in-session, and after repeated readings, I could not get past page two without weeping. His testimony to the healing he experienced overcame all his straight-arrow beliefs about 'party drugs', and his essay showed clearly the decisive action and gentle power of this medicine. This work can only authentically be described by the individuals who have

exposed themselves to it, and who may subsequently feel impelled to
share their good fortune with others.

When I sat before the trio of doctors, after undergoing extensive testing for insomnia and related sleep disorders, the diagnosis was unanimous. The kind female MD, a few years younger than I, stated with certainty, "You have Post-Traumatic Stress Disorder, PTSD."

"What?" I responded, not even really knowing what this was. "How do you know? How did I get it?"

"You've been in a war," she said. "A different kind of war, but a war, nevertheless."

When I had first entered the sleep centre a few weeks before, I knew I had to do something. I was driving and my hands were shaking off the wheel. I was bleary-eyed from nights, months, even years of not sleeping properly, and I was having trouble focusing on the road. A few weeks earlier, I noticed I was having difficulty completing sentences, finding them trailing off into nothingness and nonsense when I spoke to a friend or client. People had remarked I wasn't looking particularly well, but I went on with a dismissal and a tube of under-eye concealer. What was happening? I knew I had been dealing with all sorts of things that had crept up over the years, putting them in some subconscious file to be examined later, when I had the time. But time wasn't on my side, and when I realised I was probably endangering pedestrians or other drivers, that was it.

I was fortunate to live near a town with a sleep disorders' clinic, and within a week, I was having a consultation. When first interviewed, you are asked for any reasons you might know for your insomnia. "Well," I said, "I had a lot of death in my life, and that sort of started the whole thing, but everybody has death in their life, right?" I was forty-seven-years old at the time, and I thought losses occurred to a person in middle age. The doctors listened and said they would like to put me into a sleep study group. "Why not?" I said, "Anything could help."

So, within a week or so, and for two weeks thereafter, I entered the hospital at eight in the evening and had what seemed like a hundred electrodes hooked up to my head and body. Then I was placed into a nice little bedroom. It resembled a motel—bland, clean, and non-descript, except for a camera observing me all night long. For someone having sleeping problems, this is NOT the way to go, I thought. But, strangely enough, I got to sleep (as much as I was sleeping anywhere) and was observed and recorded. This study was to rule out any physiological reasons for sleeplessness, such as apnoea and restless leg syndrome. None of that for me...too easy. I went back to the doctors' office, and then the questioning began.

"When did this start?" asked one physician.

"Oh, maybe eight or ten...maybe eleven years ago," I said.

"What happened then?" she asked.

"Oh, well," I began hyperventilating, "I had a lot of people dying in my life, and it was difficult," I replied.

"Why were they dying?" she asked.

"Well, you see, I am a gay man, and, uh, well, aside from the 'normal' deaths one has, older relatives, favourite teachers etc., so many of my friends had AIDS, and they needed care. It was so terrible.

Then, the floodgates opened.

"It just didn't stop," I said. "One friend would get sick and then another, and I was in hospitals and nursing homes a few times a week for the last ten or twelve years, and it just went on and on and on. I couldn't recover from one when another would get cytomegalovirus (CMV), or Kaposi's Sarcoma (KS), or I heard that someone I knew had just jumped out a window. And there was no help, because the Gay Men's Health Crisis centre was overwhelmed, and Ronald Reagan wasn't allocating any funds. We all thought we would get sick if we even touched our friends who needed help."

I don't know when this outpouring ended, but I know when I looked up at these doctors and saw such pain on their gentle faces, I thought, oh, God, they're looking at me, and this is what they see: Pain. I was certainly feeling it as I spoke and sobbed more. This wasn't like me. I am an adult, child of an alcoholic; I know what is worth crying about, and what isn't; I don't need any special attention; I am here, functioning, and ready for anything. I've got armour created years ago, and nobody sees life get the best of me. But, this wasn't life; this was death, and death and I weren't really acquainted. Not until now.

When I settled down a bit and focused on what I heard myself saying, I began chronicling the events of the previous twenty years. In the beginning of the eighties, when I first went to New York to be an actor, I was invited to a small party on the Upper

East Side. A gay couple lived there, friends of friends, and it was full of actors and artists. I remember thinking, this is where gay men and women can be comfortable and at home. This is what New York City gave you—a haven, a place to work and play, where gay people could have fine and respectable lives and businesses woven into the main fabric of everyday life and society. In New York, and especially in the arts, being gay had long ceased to be an issue, but something new and frightening was brewing. I noticed a small quiet conversation in a corner of the railroad flat and walked over to join in.

"What's going on, gents? You all look too serious," I asked.

One of the hosts looked dourly at me and said, "We're talking about the gay cancer."

A shudder went through me. I shook off the remark with habitual alacrity but the feelings remained. "What do you mean, 'gay cancer'? That's impossible."

"It's happening," the host said. "Gay men are getting sick and dying, nobody is talking about it, and no one knows why or what's going on."

I was new to this scene, hearing talk of the opera, the theatre, museums, Fire Island, and now, just an hour or so after being introduced to this new species, the conversation shifted to the cancer that only afflicted gay men. I couldn't shake those shudders.

Time passed. I was lucky enough to begin working very quickly in the theatre and was out of town much of the time with show after show. I heard about the gay disease occasionally on the road, but because I was away so often, most of the news I received was from the press, and that was almost nonexistent. Until 1983, when the cover of *Newsweek* came out with a defiant gay couple on the cover and it read: Gay America, Sex, Politics, and the Impact of AIDS.

There was no denying it now. Gay men were getting sick by the thousands nationwide, and still no one knew the cause.

By this time, I had made some solid friendships in the New York theatre. When one of us would return home from a job or show, we would all have dinner together to catch up on current events. We were all so giddy to trade war stories of life on the road. But my dear friend, Paul, was developing a cough, and Craig, a sturdy, handsome twenty-six-year-old actor I had met at an Equity Library Theatre production, disappeared soon after the show ended, and no one could find him. Rick, a friend I had met through Paul, went home to visit his parents in Oregon and never returned. My cute new acquaintance, Christopher, couldn't stop the night sweats and was having uncontrollable diarrhoea. Julie's brother, Danny, died of some brain disease, and no one could explain it. Most of these men were no more than thirty years old.

Then, the apocalypse began; the lack of support and government funding to abate the crisis enabled the virus to spin out of control. No one knew how this virus was transmitted, and everyone was afraid of it. Without a government policy or doctrine, everyone was floundering for an answer.

Some health care professionals and clinics wouldn't care for these men. The emergency rooms were full of young men wasting away, their bodies attacked by dark red KS bruises, many quickly going blind from CMV and suffocating from pneumocystis pneumonia. With the ever-spiralling spread of the disease, no prescribed method of treatment, and death from a horrible set of opportunistic infections, the victims didn't know where to turn or what to do. Young infected men were throwing themselves in front of trains and off buildings.

The disease, itself, was unspeakable, but the stigma attached to it was equally heinous. These once young, healthy, and beautiful young men who walked the NYC streets now looked like Holocaust victims, with wasted and grey faces, emaciated bodies, and sunken, hollowed-out eyes, attached to oxygen machines and precariously balancing on canes and walkers. The level of fear, paranoia and judgement cast upon them was only equalled by the voraciousness of the virus that was tearing their bodies apart. People shunned them, crossed the city streets to avoid walking near them and averted their gaze. The cordial handshake was avoided, and the occasional hug on the street between friends and acquaintances was polarising. Once ill, many of these men were not welcomed back home, cast out by their families who were unfamiliar with New York life, homosexuality, and, above all, AIDS. The few recently created support groups were all overburdened and saturated with thousands of infected men needing help, and the wards and emergency rooms of hospitals who would take them were overwhelmed. These men had nowhere to turn, except to their friends, and many of us were also ill or becoming ill quickly.

But not all of us. Not me.

That is when the personal deluge of death began for my partner and I, and it was coming at us from all sides. Our first friend to contract the virus was a married father of two children under the age of three. His wife, an old friend of mine, called me one day, and after stumbling when I asked the normal questions, like "How is everything, how are the kids, and how is Bill?" she blurted out, "Uhhh...Bill is sick. Oh, Carl, he has AIDS."

And, so began our journey into the world of plastic gloves and syringes, the medical waste containers outside the apartment doors, the fumbled trips to the besieged doctors, the quest for experimental treatment from Paris and Mexico, the calls in the middle of the night, the incessant coughing, the KS lesions appearing everywhere, the diarrhoea, the soaked sheets from urine and perspiration, and the fear...the uncharted propulsion of fear.

In the middle of this plague, my dear friend, Paul, asked me to be his medical proxy when his time came to exit this world. He felt that his beloved partner, John (who became symptomatic two weeks after Paul's death and died two years later, after a series of agonising illnesses), would not be able to make the decision to help end his life when the time came. He was right. The last few days of Paul's brave battle were filled with tears, screams, and pain. When the hospice worker walked in, Paul collapsed in recognition of the implication, and as he drifted into a comatose state, I collapsed with fatigue having been up for over thirty-six hours straight watching him closely, with the nurse and the morphine pump at hand.

"Just a little sleep," I said to myself. "Just a little to give me strength to get me through these next few hours." I lay my head down in the adjoining guest room, next to the living room where Paul lay waiting to die. As I tried to quiet myself, I heard Paul's laboured breathing, and yet I had to sleep just a bit…to prepare myself for the worst, to brace myself; and, yes, to escape.

As I awoke, I heard a sound the nurse described as the "death rattle," signalling death is imminent.

"How could I?" I said to myself, "How could I dare sleep, when he lay dying in the next room?"

How dare I, quite. That is where it all began.

So, that night at Paul's home in Montauk in 1994 when he died, so did my sleep. It didn't happen all at once, but came along with the other symptoms of PTSD; wincing at triggers like the sound of someone walking down the street with an irregular gait, the snapping of any plastic mimicking the sound of rubber gloves being fitted on the hand, the smell of a hospital room, or the everyday winter cough that reminds me of someone uncontrollably drowning in their own fluid. These would elicit shaking, breathlessness, and quiet spasms, and I would bolt somewhere and attempt to compose myself.

As I explained to the doctors, there was virtually no recovery time between illnesses and death. They overlapped like waves and, also like the sea, they were perpetual and torrential. As younger people, then in our thirties, we hadn't yet developed the equipment that helps prepare us for death as we mature and get older. For most of us, the expected losses gradually begin with a grandparent or parent. It was primordial, but not in this case. This was abhorrent, as are all plagues, I suppose; and we were working in unchartered territory with an undeveloped set of tools, just flailing about for help, for medication and prayers.

Now, I am told I have PTSD, and, predictably, survivor guilt. To deal with the massive deaths of my friends is bad enough, but to go deep into my psyche where the guilt lives is more than I can bear on a daily basis. But, due to some wonderful medical professionals, friends, and loved ones, I am learning to try.

So, I went to another appointment, where I would investigate another treatment for this condition that has haunted me and kept me awake; there is new hope for me, yet from a most strange and foreign therapy. A dear friend put me in touch with a close, close friend of hers, a medical doctor who specialises in trauma. When we spoke on the phone, he mentioned MDMA as a possibility for treatment.

After a brief conversation, during which he listened to the litany of my treatments over the years, he remarked, "Well, you've certainly done it all. Would you be willing to try this?" I responded quickly with, "I will try anything. You are my last hope." Although I only knew this man through our few phone calls and emails, and mostly through my friend, whom I both loved and trusted, I decided to take a deep breath, do some research, and move forward. I took his advice and did copious research on the web, where I found such a wealth of material that I was quickly overwhelmed. I read as much as I could digest, and within a few weeks, he called.

"Well, Carl, I have found someone who can administer the MDMA and guide you through the sessions."

I gulped, and asked my final question:

"I am naïve to these substances, but most of the reading I did refers to this as a party drug, and that is just not my style. I trust you implicitly and am desperate for relief, but it sounds scary."

He responded deftly with compassion and clarity:

"Trust me, Carl, I wouldn't be pointing you toward this if you didn't sound like a perfect candidate, and the people who are helping people like you are at great risk, so believe me, this is no party drug. And the experience for you will probably be very intense, because of the pain and long trauma you have endured, but I truly believe this could bring you some relief. Many medical professionals have been experimenting with this drug, because of the veterans coming back from Iraq, and the results have been astonishing. But nobody can make this decision for you, and I am here to help if you decide to go forward."

I took the number of the person he gave me and made the call.

Within a week, I met Archie, my new friend and MDMA practitioner, who explained the process to me, how the medicine reacts chemically, how I would likely feel during the six-hour session, and, hopefully, the enlightenment, relief, and healing it might provide. We met for the consultation in his beautiful, old, and stalwart home, surrounded by layers of books, artworks, and fabrics from years of travelling and collecting. I immediately felt relaxed and secure.

On the day of the session, I took the prescribed dose, donned the eyeshades, lay back and waited.

Time has no place here. It is suspended as I fall deeper and deeper into what can only be described as the place where the pain lives, and it rushes up through me. I have acute visions of all my friends and loved ones who have died, pushing from inside me, yet out of me, as they too are desperate to be released. I cry and scream with relief and fear that they are leaving forever. Yet, I know intuitively that this is exactly what must occur in order to set me free. I plead, "I love you, I am so sorry I wasn't there for all of you, please forgive me, but you must let me sleep. Please forgive me, but you must let me sleep. Please let me sleep."

Archie holds my hand and cradles me as I cry, scream, and purge. I realise more and more that under conventional therapies, I may have never reached these dark areas where the trauma has lodged—the memories, the sadness, the guilt, the loss of these nearly twenty years of my life. They have been locked out of my daily consciousness, and as a means of survival, I have hidden them far from sight. But now it is time to face them, the memories and the loved ones, and, hopefully, release them.

But I can't let them go. This is where my friends live, and I, as penance for surviving, must bear witness, for if they live in me, they will not be forgotten, and their lives will have meant something. But, I must release them. I cannot continue to lead a half-life of never truly being awake, and never truly being asleep. As I lay heaving and wrenching with the pain of their pain, and the searing visions of what they endured, Archie says, "Let them go, Carl. Let them go. They don't want you to live this way. They want you to be free and healthy. Let them go. They are at peace, Carl, they are at peace."

And for the first time, I hear these words and know they are true. I look up and see them all unleashed from my soul, where I have protected them. As they begin to drift away from me, smiling and shimmering with youth as they once were, they say "Thank you," and I let them go—Christopher, and John, and Bobby, and Joe, and Paul, and Alex, and Dennis, and Lenny, and Danny and Sal, and Steve, and Richard, and Malcolm, and Nick, and Craig, and Rob, and Jimmy, and Gary, and Jay, and Michael, and Glenn, and Stu and, and, and...And, I wonder how many men like me wander the streets of the city seeing the dead walk beside them? And, I breathe, and the heaving subsides, and I say to Archie, "Can I sleep a little bit?" and he smiles knowingly, covers me over with a warm blanket and lets me fall finally, peacefully, and soundly, asleep.

When I awoke from this sleep within the session, I was, needless to say, wrung out. I remembered most of it, but the feeling was like the lifting of a weight. It's as though my chest (and heart) had been bound and wrapped tight with this agony, and now, the band holding it down had been released, stretched, and shattered. Archie looked at me, as he did throughout the session, sitting vigil, giving warmth and reassurance that what had happened needed to happen.

"How do you feel?" he asked.

I said, "Exhausted, weary, tired, but lighter. But I slept, didn't I? I remember sleeping soundly like I haven't slept in years."

"Yes," he replied, "toward the end of the session, you slept. You needed to, my friend. That was a rough experience. There was so much there, Carl, that you needed to get out, and you did a great deal of work toward that end."

I left that day knowing something momentous had happened. I

knew there had been a fundamental shift in my being, and it felt like nothing I had ever felt before. I was wobbly, but understood I had met and addressed a deep, deep part of my being. This was where the trauma had lived and been stored, and I had never known how to reach it before. But MDMA didn't just *allow* me that reach; it brought it forth and *made it possible* for me to face the experience of loss and pain. It's as though the medicine knew it was there to heal me. Like an antibiotic attacking a germ, or a surgeon finding the diseased organ, it recognised the source of the pain and unleashed it, because it knew it was the only way the healing could begin. PTSD prevents you from recognising the trauma, because it believes the psyche cannot handle it. MDMA trusts the body and recognises it *must* be recognised to be released. And that is exactly how my healing began.

Over the next few years, I had more sessions, all of which I approached with some nervousness but trusting in the outcome. The trauma had been forthright and ferocious that first session, but as the sessions went on, the pain gradually subsided, the memory of my loving friends became incorporated into my daily life. Less and less sleepless nights, no more visitations, just memories I can live with, and almost cherish, as one typically does with loved ones who have died.

The sessions presented themselves in a strange and magical way: As time went on and the trauma and the memories faded, the image in my mind was of a large white room, where all my friends had been housed (and trapped, I suppose) in my consciousness. During the sessions, I would approach the door to this room with trepidation, because I knew it was filled with pain. Then, gradually, over several months, somewhere in the sixth session, I approached the door and finally turned the handle. I was petrified of what lay inside, but as I opened the door, I saw an empty room, clean, bright, and white, and free of the beloved friends and all the pain that accompanied them. I remember saying in the session, "There is no more pain...no more pain."

And I knew, then, that I was free.

In that same session, I met my 'guide,' a benevolent presence that has been with me since I was a child living in a cacophonous alcoholic household. Once, when the vibration in my home was reaching the point of no return, it told me, "You won't have to live here forever." This supportive presence had remained with me my entire life, and although I recognised the voice, I had never seen the being. But there it was, devoid of gender, smiling and bringing forth a dear older friend whom I had loved and cherished. She was saying all is well, and we all live in beauty and peace. The MDMA had been a beautiful conduit. And then, once again, I slept.

I returned several times thereafter, because I discovered, although the trauma was gone, I needed to learn how to sleep properly again. During one of my sleep centre experiences, a technician had explained when chronic insomnia occurs, the unconscious begins to recognise this poor sleep pattern as the true pattern, and therefore the disturbed sleep pattern is all the body knows. But I began to discover that when I slept in my MDMA sessions, it was a deep and relaxing sleep like I hadn't known in years. The sessions just naturally became more about my peaceful sleeping and waking four to ten hours later with a restful and restorative feeling. I asked Archie, "Is it possible that because my body doesn't house the trauma anymore, the MDMA is helping me re-graph my sleeping pattern because that too needs healing?"

"It's possible," he replied. "It is a remarkable medicine." Instinctively, I knew that was what was happening, and I just laid back and let the wonder in.

Now, I am doing very well. My sleep is sound; I live with the beautiful memories in a safe and sacred place, and I have restored balance to my life. I do go back from time to time as a "tune up" as I call it, and now I sleep almost entirely through the whole session, knowing I am still creating a template of sleep I can depend upon.

In one of my last sessions, my 'guide' appeared for a second time. As I looked at the sweet, smiling face and expressed my gratitude for all the years of guidance and love, the being smiled knowingly and beatifically and said, "We are all here together, the living and the dead." I saw my life full of all those who are here and all those who are gone, walking side-by-side, hand in hand, and I smiled.

And, I slept.

Carl's first session was peopled by many un-embodied souls and overwhelmed him in the best way, enabling the release of an enormous piece of his anguished mix of fear, guilt, and regret that he had carried for twenty years. This releasing continued over time as he returned to the work, and true to the medicine's form, his subsequent sessions became less and less intense. He found in continued sessions an effective means to correct the psychic disturbances expressed as symptoms, in his case insomnia and erratic sleep patterns. The body knows what it needs and, as demonstrated here, will heal itself when given half a chance. Following the release of the traumatic core of his dysfunction, Carl slept in sessions and joyfully celebrates this recovered skill. Today, he continues his involvement as a theatre actor and works as a volunteer in a neighbouring hospice.

NON-ORDINARY CONSCIOUSNESS
AND THE TRANSPERSONAL REALM

"Our normal waking consciousness, rational consciousness as we call it, is but one special type of consciousness, while all about it, parted from it by the filmiest of screens, there lie potential forms of consciousness entirely different."

WILLIAM JAMES

We live our lives in ordinary consciousness and may pay little heed to other states, perhaps even dismissing them as "spacing out" or "daydreaming," believing they are of no value. The fact is non-ordinary states of consciousness are a part of our evolutionary legacy, a faculty we maintain after millions of years of development from primates to man. If this faculty was of no use to us, the capacity to enter non-ordinary consciousness itself would have fallen away aeons ago. However, what are they, and what is their evolutionary function?

Dreams are likely the non-ordinary state with which we are most familiar, and they arrive when our controlling ego self is asleep. Freud called them, "the royal road to the unconscious," and from his work with nitrous oxide, his American contemporary William James described the shift from ordinary to non-ordinary in the quote above.

It is indeed "all about us," and work with MDMA creates a vast expansion of our consciousness for a few precious hours by flooding the brain with serotonin. This expansion is, itself, non-ordinary, a state of being quite beyond our capacity to conjure up from ordinary consciousness. It is the experiences and insights that come to us from within this condition, articulated in many testimonies, that demonstrably attests to their value and utility.

MDMA experiences first engage with biographical material that contains elements, particularly traumatic ones, which we need to deal with by allowing their examination and release. The expansion of consciousness created by MDMA, however, may continue beyond any earthbound events to become transpersonal, literally beyond the personal, a non-ordinary state conditioned by nothing except its own capacity for boundlessness. Some of the testimonies describe experiences that fall into this realm and can be taken at face value, even as they may give pause to our credulity. The final testimony in this book is an example of an experience with MDMA that is almost entirely transpersonal.

Our interpretation of the outcomes from this work is that they bear witness to the inestimable value of non-ordinary consciousness, up to and including the transpersonal realm.

In This Book

"Perhaps the greatest gift one can give to another human being is not any thing, not ideas, not knowledge, but one's full attention."

KRISHNAMURTI

Strong experimental evidence supports the promise we find in MDMA. In this book, we will look at the research, focusing on clinical trials by Michael Mithoefer, M.D., et al. and published in peer-reviewed journals. MDMA's reputation has been tarnished from being identified only as a party drug and is virtually unknown as a medicine with considerable healing potential. The empirical research now beginning to appear is a vital countervailing force to this limited view. We will talk about ways to separate fact from fiction and provide resources readers can pursue to gain more knowledge on their own.

The central purpose of this book is, however, to examine the healing potential of MDMA through the testimonies of clients who have experienced the healing potential of this medicine. These come from a wide range of individuals beset with a broad spectrum of conditions. Through this lens, readers can feel something of what it's like to experience the medicine work and understand the necessity of the presence of an attendant throughout a client's session. Being present for the client experiencing MDMA is crucial to this work; as attendants, we are like parents sitting with a sick child, or doulas supporting the birthing process. We are not healing anyone or making anything happen; we are simply present, very present.

"If you really love that person and want to help them, be with them. Sit with them. You don't have to talk. You don't have to do anything. But really be there."

ELIZABETH KUBLER-ROSS

Introduction

"But such is the irresistible nature of truth, that all it asks, and all it wants is the liberty of appearing."

THOMAS PAINE

From our experience, we feel an obligation to act on our understanding that we already possess the medicine we need to release trauma: MDMA. To take maximum advantage, we need to respect this medicine by standing back, making a deep bow, and acknowledge the deep psychic opening it makes possible by letting it do its work in facilitating the release of traumatic material captured by the body. The clinical evidence to support that claim will be addressed in Chapter One, but first, let's consider the optimum context for this work.

BUILDING TRUST

Any therapeutic process aimed at healing trauma (or anything else) begins with a trusting relationship, known as the "therapeutic alliance." In orthodox interpersonal therapeutic practice, the client seeks help from a therapist who brings authority, knowledge, and insight to the table. The client needs to know the therapist is trustworthy, objective, completely on their side, and has their best interests at heart. If that relationship can be established, therapy can progress and hopefully bear fruit.

With MDMA, creating the therapeutic alliance is arguably even more important. A client under the influence of the medicine needs a trustworthy attendant at least as much as a client in conventional therapy. In this work, the clients may feel especially vulnerable. They wear eyeshades and lie in a prone position which can, itself, induce feelings of helplessness. Embarking upon what is essentially an inner journey, the client needs to know they can trust the therapeutic alliance established between themselves and their attendant. It is crucial the client knows everything that happens in the therapy room will be to their benefit, and nothing will happen they do not want to happen.

MDMA may be a particularly valuable tool for establishing the therapeutic alliance in any context as it lowers anxiety, fear, and the dark, negative ideas we have about ourselves. Feeling complete trust in the alliance we have established, we can enter the session with equanimity and ease.

LOOKING BEYOND SYMPTOMS

"There are no limits to the depths to which the mind will go to deceive itself."

ANNE OTHER

All meaningful work in non-ordinary conscious is intra-psychic. The conversation is within us, and all other actors are irrelevant to the unfolding that occurs.

The interpersonal talk therapy format puts certain boundaries on our experience by requiring the client to verbalise everything. The therapist responds in kind based on his or her analysis of thoughts offered up by the client per their training. It is a cognitive method that can lead to useful insights, but critically, it fails to fully engage one essential element of human psychology, feelings, and emotional expression.

Consider our self-definition: Homo sapiens, the thinking human. We enthusiastically embrace Descartes' most famous saying, "I think, therefore I am," as the whole truth, when it is, in fact, only partial. A wiser and more complete self-description would be Homo sapiens *et affectus*; the thinking and feeling human. Such a readjustment to our identity is not uncommon from exposure to our deeper selves in this medicine work.

Focusing on the cognitive at the expense of the emotional is normal in today's world. If you ask someone how they are feeling, they will likely say something generic, like, "I am doing OK," but seldom much in the way of specifics. We just do not tend to give the same weight or value to our feelings that we do to our thoughts. It is an unfortunate bias.

Cognitive integration is an essential and valuable element of this medicine work. So much information comes up in each session that most people come away with new thoughts, feelings, and realisations that may require time to digest. Following their medicine sessions, clients work with a therapist, spiritual leader, or other skilled practitioner to talk about ways to best utilise this new knowledge in their lives.

However, such cognitive interpersonal work using words, discussing concepts and thoughts and ideas and so on, is inappropriate in the MDMA session room. Instead, we provide the maximum opportunity for the medicine to reveal to the client the true depth, breadth, and height of their psyche by doing nothing ourselves. We do not guide or lead the client in any way. Conversations are kept to a necessary minimum. Of course, we respond when spoken to, but primarily, we are there simply as attendants, offering a hand to hold, a glass of water or an extra blanket, as human beings, not as therapists. In essence, the less we do, the more the medicine can do.

Instead of seeing symptoms as messengers trying to alert us to the underlying situation, allopathic medicine seeks to eliminate the symptoms themselves. Psychological and psychopharmacological approaches follow this logic. They ask, "Do you feel depressed? Okay, take this medicine; you won't feel so depressed anymore." Meanwhile, you may not feel much of anything at all anymore. The treatment is essentially reductive. MDMA therapy, on the other hand, is fundamentally expansive. The medicine experience enlarges and broadens your worldview, putting you directly in touch with the feeling part of yourself.

GOING INSIDE

Whatever the location, the MDMA session room promotes access to deep emotions. It is a pure, uncluttered space, often in the client's home or where they feel most comfortable. They can simply sink into themselves. We say, "You have nothing to do. Just lie back and allow the medicine to approach you." The session offers an environment where it is safe to surrender to the medicine in preparation for receiving whatever is revealed without fear or favour. Rather than numbing and separating them from their internal experience, this work allows clients to meet and engage with their traumas as part of themselves.

All of us working on this book have had that meeting with our deepest selves. Here is a little more about one attendant's background, how she came to the medicine, and why she feels compelled to share its gifts with others:

"The root source of my own dysfunction was my mother's death in the closing months of World War II; I was two months old. My family was thrown into trauma and chaos, and I was looked after by my maternal grandmother and others. My aunt came to take care of me and my two-year-old brother two months later, when she was released from her nursing obligations at the end of the war. Upon meeting me for the first time, she said I was "stiff as a board," expressing nothing.

At school, I was diagnosed with a cognitive deficit on account of showing zero ability in mathematics, forward thinking or conceptualisation, while excelling in other areas. I was very, very shy and suffered all my life from chronic social anxiety. I attended college, pursued art and took up teaching in London. Everything looked normal. My early traumas, however, had stayed with me.

During my teaching days, suddenly, I just broke down. I was working three and a half days a week, but for the rest of the week, when I should have been developing a freelance practice, I could not get out of bed. I just lay there in a fetal position. I could not even answer the phone. I had no idea what to do; I was completely naïve about psychology at this point. I was completely exhausted and thought it might be a lack of iron. I never even entertained the idea that my mother's passing would have affected me all these years later. I thought I had grown up in a perfectly normal, loving family, which we were in every way but for this tragedy. The thing was, as a family, we never truly acknowledged, let alone grieved, this shattering event. Even mentioning my mother was simply too painful for my father to bear, so we did not. The greatest presence in our home was the absence of our mother.

Fortunately, a friend gave me Arthur Janov's just-published book, *The Primal Scream*, and I devoured it. It was like reading the innermost pages of my mind, pages I had never even had access to before. Janov not only described how I was feeling, but offered a way to ameliorate it. He demonstrated that if you had a severe trauma when you were young, the traumatic events were going to have a knock-on effect throughout your life. Through primal therapy, he suggested, you can address and express that trauma.

Reading that book gave me the information I needed to be able to accept my situation. I vigorously pursued primal therapy, and little by little, I expanded my emotional range, which had been essentially nonexistent; I experienced myself as an outline. Anger was the most accessible. I could realise the rage and, by expressing it, was eventually able to experience and feel the hurt behind the rage. I could shout, scream, and weep. For the first time, I had contact with my feeling self.

I encountered another somatic method of processing trauma, Stanislav Grof's breathwork, around twenty years later. Grof had conducted research with psychoactive substances in the 1950s and 1960s, before prohibition, so he understood the larger picture of the psyche. Primal therapy rejoined me with my ability to feel. Breathwork greatly expanded my awareness of what was possible by including the spiritual dimension.

Over time, I became more aware and informed about MDMA's potential as a healing agent; I had no interest in it as a party drug. I approached someone I trusted and asked her to sit with me. I went to her house, somewhat anxious. Being cut off from the memory of the things I had experienced was no longer serving me. Something had to change.

The session itself was absolutely marvellous. My sitter, Maria, was patient and kind, and her quiet, centred, and gracious behaviour has become the model for us attendants. I took the MDMA, and it was simply a revelation. I entered a state of vastly expanded consciousness about who I was and who I could be; it was exactly what I needed. I found myself in a safe cocoon of loving, hopeful feelings for myself and others. I had always been intense, tightly wound like the bands that make up a golf ball. With the medicine, these bands simply let go. Within that relaxed space, I was free to meet and engage with the greater part of the trauma I had suffered.

I was away from home for this first session, and I had to go back home the next day on a train. Previously, I had always been anxious with strangers. Not this day. I was with a group of people in the train carriage, and it was just the sweetest thing; I tear up, whenever I recall it. The whole carriage seemed to be in a relaxed and beautiful mood that I became part of and enjoyed with them. I had been released from the worst of my social anxiety. I realised, "Oh, this has *already* changed my actual life!" Never mind the experience of the session itself, which was remarkable; I found myself a truly changed woman the next day and for the days thereafter.

After this stunning event, I was never again troubled in the same way by the social anxiety that had plagued me all my life. My anxiety was extreme enough that I had significant trouble entering a room full of strangers and was a wallflower at every gathering I attended. After this single MDMA session, my extreme anxiety was reduced to normal levels. I was astonished. The effect would have been lovely if it had lasted only a short while, but I have never slid back into that debilitating level of anxiety. The outcome has maintained unto this day."

In addition to its ability to release us from trauma, the potential for lasting change with MDMA really impressed me. Over time, the notion of sharing with others the healing potential I had found took hold. I came to work with others, because I had, myself, experienced the healing potential of MDMA; my gratitude was off the charts. I started working with one or two people, then three or four, and soon enough, I met others who were doing the same work."

If we fully allow ourselves to unwind, and MDMA gives us the greatest assist imaginable in that endeavour, we can come back together better than ever. The organism knows what it needs. That is the fundamental idea behind this work. The body knows how to heal itself, and given the opportunity to do so, will do so. To our experience and observation, this medicine presents us with the most superb opportunity for enabling the body to heal itself.

CHAPTER ONE

A Brief History of MDMA

"It's not what we don't know, it's what we do know that ain't so."

MARK TWAIN

The trajectory of MDMA from patent to utility is quite well-known and available from other sources. We offer this brief account for unfamiliar readers.

When MDMA was first synthesised, nobody knew quite what it was or what to do with it. Merck Pharmaceutical had developed the compound in Germany before World War 1 and had been granted a patent in 1914, but they had no idea what its possible applications or utility might be. It remained on the shelf until 1918 when Germany had lost the war and to the victors went the spoils. Pharmaceuticals and other items were divvied up as part of war reparations. Thus, MDMA arrived in the United States, where Dow Chemical searched for a way to use it. Like Merck before them, however, Dow was also at a loss as to what to make of this compound.

One organic chemist, however, Alexander Shulgin, was very curious about MDMA and was given, by Dow, the rights to work with this substance that both they and Merck had considered worthless. With an adventurous spirit and a laboratory of his own, Shulgin pressed on. While working with the compound, he ingested some himself and found it to have remarkable effects.

As a lay-therapist, his wife, Ann Shulgin, quickly saw MDMA's potential for enabling people who were "stuck" in their recovery from trauma and other depredations to become open to more of their inner psychic material than could be brought forth through talking in a traditional counselling session. MDMA radically expanded the subconscious material available to the client's consciousness.

In the 1970s and 1980s, therapeutic medicine work by people like

Ann Shulgin and psychotherapist, Leo Zeff, helped demonstrate MDMA's potential, and word spread rapidly. Zeff, a Bay Area psychotherapist, was so impressed by the healing potential of the medicine that he came out of retirement to hold MDMA gatherings at his house. An anonymous book, *The Secret Chief,* described his methods, and after his death, a second book, *The Secret Chief Revealed*, was published with Zeff's name on it.

Out of the work by people like the Shulgins and Leo Zeff, a community of therapists developed around the use of MDMA. They and other counsellors offered it to their clients in various ways to promote an expansion of the psyche that allowed for accelerated progress in trauma recovery and psychological healing.

FIRST IMPRESSIONS

Word of MDMA's euphoria-inducing effects spread widely into the community at large, and related compounds made their way into the non-therapeutic community. On the party scene, a recreational product called "ecstasy" became ubiquitous. The problem with ecstasy, as opposed to pure MDMA, is it is frequently adulterated in ways that can harm the user. The products pushed at raves have a very sketchy reputation as drugs that make people fall, overheat, overhydrate, and end up in the Emergency Room or worse. What is most often happening, though, is ravers get hold of seriously contaminated products that can wreak havoc on their bodies. One recent incident involved a man who was sold something called MDMA, though it actually contained 60 percent caffeine and 40 percent MDA, a relative of MDMA with different properties. It was like ingesting a pack of Lucozade Energy or Red Bull! That is not the MDMA experience we are talking about.

Other problems tarnished the drug's reputation, such as the precipitous post-dose drop in serotonin levels that can be problematic without the proper support. Emergency Room (ER) personnel may see patients with this syndrome after big party weekends. A person who uses ecstasy on a Saturday night may show up in the ER on the following Tuesday, because they have burned through their amino acid stores and are not producing enough new serotonin. Some ER folks with a dark sense of humour call it, "Suicide Tuesday," because these patients are depressed beyond belief.

When emergency situations precipitated by *ecstasy* and its ilk became more frequent on the streets, alarm bells went off. It appeared as if MDMA was unsafe and unpredictable, even though the product they ingested was not pure MDMA but the adulterated product—ecstasy. In addition, people who thought they were ingesting MDMA did not know what was in the *ecstasy* they were taking, so they could not know how to take it safely. Legislators, social workers, and parents were concerned and wanted to get ecstasy off the streets, while the therapeutic community knew that 100 percent pure, medical grade MDMA was both safe and extraordinarily useful.

Unfortunately, the scheduling of MDMA by the US Drug Enforcement Agency (DEA) turned out to be heavily influenced by fear of the drug. Originally slated for Schedule I classification in 1984, rendering the drug illegal even for therapeutic purposes, MDMA got a stay of execution when therapists requested administrative hearings. Judge Francis Young listened to the testimonies and ruled on the issue, coming down with a decision worthy of Solomon—he split it right down the middle. He ruled MDMA be designated a Schedule III drug, available to researchers and for prescription by psychiatrists. The victory was short-lived, however; the subsequent ruling by the DEA has placed MDMA on Schedule 1 since 1985, out of the reach of those who need it most.

This ruling, in place for the past thirty-two years, was described as temporary. It is our hope this volume may support efforts to return to Judge Young's judicial decision to place MDMA on Schedule III.

CLINICAL TRIALS

"You will observe with concern how long a useful truth may be known and exist before it is generally received and practised on."

BENJAMIN FRANKLIN

Fortunately, some stalwart researchers have begun research work with MDMA to prove its efficacy. Chief among them is Dr. Michael Mithoefer who, with colleagues, published the results of their Phase 1 trial entitled, "The safety and efficacy of ±3,4-methylenedioxymethamphetamine-assisted psychotherapy in subjects with chronic, treatment-resistant PTSD: the first randomised controlled pilot study" in 2010. They examined the effects of MDMA therapy on survivors of domestic violence, sexual abuse, and rape. People in these categories filled twenty slots in the study; two military veterans joined as well. The subjects were all treated with MDMA, and the results were truly impressive: Mithoefer reported an 83 percent remission of PTSD symptoms among test subjects.

Mithoefer's results were so far out of the ballpark compared to the small percentages that prove statistical significance in most studies that doubts were raised in certain quarters. Eighteen months later, once the study had been read and analysed, research scientists responded favourably, recognising it was among the most impeccable, beautifully designed and administered of studies. Mithoefer and his colleagues have since completed a Phase 2 trial with domestic abuse victims, first responders, and veterans as subjects; their results continue to be extraordinarily promising.

Next comes a Phase 3 trial, which is crucial to getting MDMA recognised as a legitimate medicine. This final leg of the research is an enormous undertaking, requiring at least 200 subjects to complete it. Subjects will be exposed to the medicine in multiple locations across the United States, Canada, and Israel, and the study aims to be completed by 2021. If everything goes as expected, an application will then be made for legalising MDMA for therapeutic use per Judge Francis Young's ruling that it be placed on Schedule III.

One of our clients, Sgt. K, is a veteran. He developed PTSD after he was wounded, and his best friend was killed next to him in an improvised explosive device (IED) explosion. He had suffered through the mayhem of war for two tours, one before 9/11 and one after.

Back home, he managed bravely. Every so often, though, he would go through a period he described as "grinding," when normal functioning became nearly impossible. For weeks on end, he forced himself out of bed, forced himself to eat breakfast, go to work, and so on.

He worked with MDMA with an attendant at the beginning of

one such depressive episode and has never had another. He has done four MDMA sessions altogether, and says he is simply done with the trauma. He goes to ballgames with his son, coaches Little League, works his job, and takes college courses. He can remember, in graphic detail, every moment of the event that traumatised him, but it no longer has the emotional charge it once had. He says he can remember it the way you remember the colour of the house you were born in. It is just another fact of life.

Yet, there is still significant resistance to the idea of using MDMA for trauma or PTSD. Sgt. K. has a hard time persuading his war buddies to try the treatment because of the "suck it up" mentality Marines are taught, and because MDMA's reputation as a party drug gives no indication of its healing potential.

Dr. Mithoefer's studies go a long way toward mitigating this negative reputation. This book includes the firsthand testimonies of dozens of clients that we hope may also serve to reveal the healing potential of MDMA.

I feel so liberated and light.

Sarah B.

*We need courage to approach this work, especially if we are afraid
the medicine may bring us to our death. Sarah was in a very dark
place in her life, but this testimony, resulting from her four sessions,
elucidates the power of MDMA to open us to the deepest parts of
our psyches that are lost to us. Her inter-generational experiences
demonstrate the medicine's ability to reveal, in astonishing detail,
the reach that is available to each and every one of us within non-
ordinary consciousness. Nothing is lost. We may have 'no memory'
of much of our past, but it all remains reachable within us through
the agency of the medicine.*

When I was told by a close friend about this MDMA work, I
must confess I was not particularly open to it. I had never done
drugs and was not the "kind of person" that needed drugs to
deal with my life. Drugs scared me, still scare me. Drugs, in my
mind, represented a loss of control and a form of escape from
something, and I never was comfortable with either. I never saw
drugs as an exploration of one's self. I saw them as an excuse to
escape one's life. But I was in a very dark place, and at a certain

point, I thought, why not? In my mind, the worst that could happen was I died, and at that point, I was willing to take that risk (like I said, I was in a dark place).

Thank goodness, I did. It was one of the best things I have ever done, and it was the beginning of an amazing journey that continues today. The medicine allowed me to explore my life in a completely unencumbered way. It allowed me to answer some of the biggest riddles of my life, and it made almost every decision I have ever made make perfect sense. My journal entry for the day following my first experience was as follows:

I have lived my life up until yesterday trying to prove that I was worthy of being born. At 11:11 a.m. I began a medicine session that allowed me to travel to all parts of my brain and to unlock moments in time that have created blocks or patterns in my life....

My journal entry goes on for pages, days actually, as more came up over the next two or three days following the experience. Everything about my first experience was pleasant. It was as if I were floating through different points in time, saw what I needed to see, understood it, and moved on. The most important observation for me that may sound totally insane for all sceptics, (and I could not have been a bigger sceptic prior) was when my mother was pregnant with me, she desperately wanted me to be a boy, and my father was sure I was going to be a boy and had even named me Jeffri. At the time, my parents' marriage was unstable, and my mother believed, if I were a boy, that my father was more likely to stay.

During my MDMA session, I felt this while in utero, and then I watched the nurse put me on my mother's chest and say, "Congratulations, it is a girl!" The first emotion I felt from my mother was disappointment. At that time, I internalised being a girl was not good enough, and I had to prove I was worthy of being born. So, I set about my life to do so. For me that meant doing "guy" things. I needed to achieve. And I did. Although I enjoyed the intellectual stimulation of what I did, it never felt quite right. I was proud of where I worked, and what I had accomplished, but it was always a grind. I put in more hours, slept less, travelled more, trying to prove what to whom, I do not know. But I felt like if I wasn't "grinding;" I was slacking, and slacking was never acceptable. Those choices make sense to me now.

I am glad I did all of that, but I feel like I now have better balance in my life as a result of my experience with the medicine. I now understand that my constant striving and the need to succeed were driven from a place of having to prove to myself that I deserved to be here, hence, no matter what I accomplished, it was never quite satisfying. Now, I am able to look at what I have done with pride. I know I am worthy. (I should note that I am still intensely ambitious, it just comes from a different place, one that is a lot more satisfying.)

During my experience, I also discovered I had absorbed various fears from both of my parents. I discovered I did not have a fear of abandonment; it was my mother's. I was never able to reconcile where that fear had come from as none of my life's experiences had led me to that. Yet, I had it anyway. That was released during my MDMA session. I had always assumed that my fear of not having money had come from my mother, as she had very little when we were growing up. However, I discovered that my fear of not having money actually came from my father. When I was born, he loved me, but felt totally trapped both in the marriage and in life as he had not yet made any money, and he was not sure how he was going to pay for my mother and me and still be able to leave the marriage. You may be thinking that my father leaving was the genesis of my abandonment issues, but bizarrely, I never felt like he left me. I always knew that he had left my mom. During the session, I released my fear of abandonment and my fear of money.

If this all sounds a little out there, it is. But I can tell you that the time I have spent doing this medicine work has had a profoundly positive and liberating impact on my life. By no means am I "cured," but the lens through which I view and interpret the world has been cleared. I still catch myself thinking, "Ooh, but that is a girl's job or too girly," or something along those lines, but now I stop myself, smile, and reassess and think: How great. Girls rule! So, my first experience was exceedingly pleasant and indeed life altering in many ways but focused primarily on this generation of my family.

Six months later, I did it again. This was a much deeper, darker experience. I do believe, although I do not know if science would back me up on this one, because I was in a much better, lighter place, I was able to handle going deeper. I went back generations this time. I released feelings of failure, unworthiness, and insecurity on behalf of my grandfathers and great-grandfathers on both sides. I observed the interactions of the marriages of my grandparents on both sides of my family, and I am dismayed to say that the dysfunction and feelings of unworthiness resembled my own marriage. Can this really happen? Can a person whose life experiences in no way would lead them to set themselves up in this way, really repeat the mistakes of their ancestors? The answer, I discovered, is clearly yes. And I did. I repeated patterns of my grandparents. It gave me a deeper, greater, and somewhat profound understanding of the demise of my marriage and my significant role in it.

So, in only two sessions, I embraced being born female, being worthy of love, actually being loved, and being able to accept help. Literally. I released "my" fear of abandonment, my father's sadness over losing his father at a young age, my confusion around money, and my need to prove that I deserved to be born. That is a big one; and the list goes on.

Following this second session, Sarah sent her attendant an e-mail, as follows:

This work is miraculous. At first, I was upset that this experience was not as positive as my last one, but what I have been able to do over the last thirty-six hours is release generations of baggage. I have released generations of sadness, feelings of failure, feelings of unworthiness, feelings of being trapped in something that I felt I was better than, and feelings that somehow the world owed me something for being good. I feel so liberated and light. It is truly miraculous. Thank you.

My third session was meant to be the closing of a chapter of my life and the opening of a new one. I did it to mark the ending of my one year of mourning my husband walking out. I had given myself that time to grieve. This time was, again, very different than the other two. For this experience, I had actually set an intention beforehand. I set out to "release all that no longer served me." It was interesting. It took me a few days to realise that is what, indeed, happened. It tied everything I had learned that year together.

But I am getting ahead of myself.

When I took the medicine this time, it affected me right away. Within a few minutes, I was watching my parents drive me home from the hospital after being born. There was very little conversation as I was strapped in the back of the car, but the messages were loud and clear. I thought, "Wow, this experience is going to be a powerful one if this is where I am starting." It was, indeed, a powerful learning experience. As for the next six and half hours, I went back to this scene over and over and over again; to the point where I tried to direct my mind to go observe something else. I remember thinking, "OK, I get it. Let's move on and let me learn something new," but instead I went back to that scene again.

The interesting thing from visiting that experience over and over again is that I was able to see it from multiple perspectives. It began with me voicing my frustration to my parents. The words, "It is not my job to take care of you; it is your job to take care of me," went through my head over and over. A five-day-old child should never feel like it is her duty to take care of others. So, I felt my pain and frustration as a newborn, and it clarified why I have always had a difficult time allowing myself to need things from anyone. I also absorbed more of my dad's fear and hope that now that I was born, my mother would finally be happy. I learned that my father was a little afraid of my mother. He had no idea how to make her happy and hoped I would be the thing that finally made her happy. There began my lifelong feeling of being responsible for my mother's happiness.

From my mother, I felt her hopes that I would be able to fix her marriage and that perhaps my dad would now stay. And there was the birth of my feeling the need to fix everything and my overwhelming feeling of responsibility for everything and everyone. I was taught at a young age that I was responsible for others, and I was not supposed to have any needs of my own. That is a lot of pressure for a newborn. I released all of that and told everyone that they were now responsible for their own happiness. It is not my job, never was.

Last and certainly not least, a little over eighteen months later, I did it again. Many things, again, were witnessed; the most poignant this time was my observing why I have always had a difficult time trusting my feelings, my happiness. So much makes sense to me now. My insecurities and neurosis make sense to me. Many of them have been released, some of them are still around and get triggered, but I am now able to look at them and observe them with perspective. I have always felt like I knew myself well, but that at the same time there was a piece I could not quite explain or reach. I reached it. I feel complete. It is remarkable. And for me, it was all thanks to the medicine work.

For many, these things may not be profound, but for me, they were life altering. In four sessions, I garnered what I deem to be a lifetime worth of therapy. My key takeaways: It is okay to be a girl, my family's history is not mine, I am not responsible for anyone else's happiness, and I can trust my own feelings. For some, those are obvious. For me, intellectually, I would say of course those things are all true, but now, thanks to MDMA, I can actually live that way. I am living my life, for me. And it feels amazing. And intensely liberating.

For Sarah to experience such events as the car ride home from the hospital where she was born (not to mention pre-natal experiences), complete with details about both her mother's and her father's feelings at that time, brings us foursquare up against reality. Really? One might imagine she had an imagination of astonishing fecundity and had invented this out of whole cloth, yet her successful outcomes tell a different story. What we see is the infinite possibility offered by transpersonal consciousness to reveal the deepest elements of the psyche. All this was made available by the action of MDMA, which gave her nothing at all in terms of content but everything in terms of making that content available to her. That availability does not end when the session ends; we are opened, and the insights may fruitfully continue for many days and weeks afterwards.

People react differently to the medicine, and this plays out in their behaviour during the session. Sarah was utterly silent and still throughout all her sessions, matching the focus that had brought success in her professional life. Her first six- to eight-hour session may have resulted in no more than two hundred words between us, and the majority of these were simple, declarative statements or questions relating to the conduct of the work. A contemplative silence is the optimal environment for making the most of this opportunity to have a meeting with ourselves.

· · ·

Our lives would have been so much different.

Dorothy.

Introduced to MDMA recreationally, Dorothy understood its power. It was not until she took the medicine in a safe environment supported by an attendant that she experienced the true depth of its healing potential.

I had known for a long time that I was unhappy, and I needed a change. A fresh start, away from all the people and situations that were causing me pain would be what I needed to find peace. Within a few short weeks, I moved across the country to start a new job in a city. Things were going well for a while, but after two years, I had not made any close relationships, and I was still unhappy, living in a perpetual cycle of anxiety and depression. Even after years of therapy, I found little satisfaction in my life. The issue wasn't everyone else; the issues were within myself.

I met a man who introduced me to MDMA. We took it recreationally. I had a deeply moving and powerful experience, gaining new insights into my life and began to question everything I believed to be true. I did not know how to process the insights. Unfortunately, without a support system to discuss my experience, I had a very difficult transition.

Over time, I noticed that I was more open to viewing the world and less judgemental of others and less judgemental of myself. I felt a new sense of urgency to return to my roots and make peace with the past. Rather than run away from my problems, I decided to return to my home city and face them head on. It was another difficult transition, returning to the problems I ran away from so many years before. There was a lot of anger about my past, and it was consuming me.

I learned about the therapeutic use of MDMA. Recalling my own past experience, I knew how powerful it could be. I wanted to have another MDMA experience; this time in a safe setting with a sitter to assist with the experience.

It was different using MDMA with an attendant in a dedicated setting. I was very anxious going to the session, not knowing what might come up from my past. The space of the attendant was so warm and inviting; it was very comforting. It put me at ease. The attendant was very compassionate and attentive, and I felt very safe. After taking the medicine, all I had to do was lay back and let the medicine do the work. Unlike talk therapy, I didn't struggle with expressing myself; with MDMA, I just had to experience the moment.

With a sense of safety, I allowed myself to go deep into my experience and my feelings. This was a new experience for me since I do NOT do feelings! One of the most powerful experiences from the session was when I heard a long-laboured exhale of a man. I heard life leave his body in his final moments and, suddenly, thoughts of my father came flowing over me. All the long-held anger that I felt for him disappeared, and I was overcome by love and compassion. I felt the love that I locked up so long ago for my father.

This scared me. Thankfully, the sitter was there for me, and I felt safe exploring the emotions more deeply. The attendant was so important in helping me integrate the experience. It's one thing to have a powerful experience, but quite another to process the information and make changes. Having a guide during the session and a support system following the experience made the transition back to everyday life more manageable.

Life has a way of throwing a curveball. Just a few days after the experience, my father was diagnosed with cancer and passed away three weeks later. I am so grateful that I had the session, because I was able to be more attentive and loving as I cared for my father during the last few weeks of his life. I will always be grateful for that time with my father. We did a lot of healing. I was able to tell my father that I loved him. In those three weeks after having this very powerful experience, I was really there for him. I can't undo all those years of anger and hatred, but we had a very meaningful three weeks. I'm very grateful for that, because who knows what those last few weeks could have been like had I not had the MDMA experience. We had a lot of very tender, sweet moments that I don't think I would have been capable of having had I not had that experience.

I had several other MDMA sessions, each with insights. I was able to heal traumas from my childhood that affected my present. Thanks to the brave and dedicated work of the attendant, I was able to experience the pain from the past with an open heart and compassion. The medicine also gave me insights to my present and showed me sides of myself that I had been blind to see. I can see life from a new lens. Change my paradigm and rewrite my story. Released from the unhealthy cycles from the past. No need to retell the old story about being broken. I can heal and move on.

It's still a work in progress, but I think things are improving. Feeling satisfaction and enjoyment was unfathomable before. Now, I can appreciate the little moments and waste less time complaining about things. I'm finding my way, and I'm getting comfortable with who I am for the first time in my life. I don't think any of that would have happened without the work with the medicine. The anxiety has improved. I am more relaxed and better able to cope with stressful situations.

It was a very positive experience, and if there was only a way that all those other people, like my father, had been able to take advantage of something like that, our lives would have been so much different.

I'm just so grateful that I found my way to it. More people need to be able to get it. It releases the darkness in us, so that we can just be ourselves.

The developmental trauma experienced by Dorothy as a child growing up with a suicidal mother, was so great that she had been unable to do meaningful work to assuage it. Perhaps the most remarkable feature of MDMA is its ability to both present us with the dark core of our dysfunction while simultaneously rendering it approachable.

It is within this action, if we are able to simply stay with the memories that emerge, the psyche has the opportunity to understand that the trauma is over and to release it. "All the anger just disappeared." Dorothy had no part in that release except, significantly, to show up for herself by offering herself to the medicine.

•   •   •

I'm not religious, but I thank God for this work.

Tawny C.

The trajectory of this young woman's work to reveal the source of her fear is a testimony to the remarkable ability of MDMA to uncover this, then that, then the other. It does not lie, and neither does it stop in its mission, and our only task in-session is to allow its inexorable progress toward the truth. It would require the creative imagination of a novelist or screenwriter to have contrived the sequence of events she uncovered, but with committed focus in every moment, she persisted until the complexity was made explicit, and she could come to understand what had happened, and how it happened. She had lived with this twisted tale mis-informing her about the most fundamental element of her relationship with her husband, his sexuality, and as the full narrative unfolds, we can see just how utterly her confusion about man-woman relationships could have arisen.

I'm going to start by saying that drugs have always terrified me. As a kid, I watched those anti-drug after-school specials, where one of the characters would take PCP and jump out the window.

I was very affected by that, and I was very anti-drugs. I even went so far as to send a letter to Nancy Reagan saying I supported the drug war.

Fast-forward to when I had to get a tooth extraction for an implant. They put me on nitrous oxide, laughing gas. I remember being on the laughing gas and having the most beautiful, spiritual experience, where I saw a white light and encountered a spirit. The spirit had two messages for me: Don't fear death, and you must do more drugs. I thought, this is so bizarre; me do more drugs? Up until then, I had no drug experience, aside from occasional marijuana. So, I was questioning this message to do more drugs. Spirit person, why must I do more drugs? At that time, a friend of mine was talking about his MDMA experiences, and I always dismissed him. I thought he was just a crazy drug-taker, and I never took him seriously at all. After my nitrous oxide experience, he mentioned it again, and I thought, "Yes! This is it! I have to do MDMA."

At this time in my life, I had just moved back to Paris from New York, and I was lost. I've never been someone that's lost, ever, in my life. I've always known exactly what I've wanted to do, and I've always been pretty cheerful. There were signs that things were not right throughout my life, like panic attacks, social anxiety, and an innate sense that something wasn't right, but I always thought that that's just me; there's nothing I'll ever be able to do about it. It's just what my life is like. I also had a lot of avoidance behaviour, and I was easily startled. I didn't understand why I had these issues, but I just figured out how to live with them.

So, when my friend mentioned MDMA again, I thought, "Okay, I'm going to take the plunge." Because a year before, I decided

I had to find ways to let go of fear. One of my major fears was spiders, so I found a way to overcome serious arachnophobia to the point that I became a fan of spiders. Now, spiders are very precious to me because that was my first step in conquering fear. I enrolled in a one-day programme to overcome my arachnophobia. The course began with talking about spiders, learning about spiders, and looking at spiders in a glass jar, and ended with holding a tarantula. I held a tarantula! And I remember feeling that it was the most beautiful creature, and how much I wanted to protect it.

I thought, wow, this is how fear works. Something that scared me so much in the end, actually saved part of me—saved me from debilitating fear. Knowing that, I thought I'd confront my fear of drugs. And after my experience with the nitrous oxide, spirit encounter, and also meeting up with my friend and him telling me about MDMA, I thought, that's it. I'm going to do something that terrifies me and conquer yet another fear.

I had no idea what to expect; I'd never even been in any sort of altered state before. Never. Alcohol, maybe, but that's so different. So, I had a lot of fear going into my first MDMA session. A lot. My fears were: Am I going to die? Am I going to be able to handle the drug? I wasn't scared of the content at all. I was scared of the possibility of death, the loss of control, and what's going to happen to me.

The morning of the session, I was nervous. I had no idea what to expect, so I just took the pill, and I lay down. I think it hit me immediately. I remember practising breathing techniques, and all of a sudden, my fingers started getting tingly, and I started getting warm and a bit sweaty.

Then, there was a moment; I felt that I was taking off on a plane going through extreme turbulence and thinking, "I can't handle this turbulence." It was just getting to be too much. And then I remember saying, "I'm overwhelmed," and my attendant said in a comforting, wonderful voice, "Just take a few breaths." I took those breaths, and then I came out of those clouds and the turbulence into the pristine, peaceful sky above the clouds, and I just thought, Aaaaaah. What a feeling. It wasn't even bliss; it was like, I'm safe. I don't need to worry anymore, I got this.

Once I reached the point of safety, I heard myself say, "Welcome, Tawny, we finally get to meet." It was my inner self finally being acquainted with my outer self. And my inner self welcomed me and said, "I've been waiting for you. We have something to discuss."

My inner self took control and took me to this room in Salt Lake City, Utah. I was immediately in that room watching myself as a four-year-old being terrorised by a family friend. I didn't know why. The question of why this happened was not revealed in the first session. All I got was what happened. I was playing around. I was being naughty; I wasn't given a clear picture of my exact behaviour, but I clearly saw him freak out at me and go into attack mode, slapping me, hitting me, and once it was over, he said, "This is our secret. We're not going to tell anybody."

I kept going back to that same scene, seeing myself being attacked over and over again. Then, at some point, I told the story out loud. I explained what happened to me, and acknowledged that it was terrifying, and that it is behind so much of my fear. Most of my panic attacks or social anxiety would happen when a tall man would be standing above me. I would go into terrible fight-

or-flight mode, for reasons I never understood. So, I realised that this relates directly to what happened to me in that room in Salt Lake City. I just remember saying, "Thank God, I found this trauma; it answers so many questions. Thank God for this work." I felt transformed; I felt like there was an unlocking of something I didn't even know existed. When I relived it in my sessions, it was like, of course this happened! How did I forget this? That was really profound for me, that I had a mechanism of blocking something like that out.

My life became so much better after that session. I felt more comfortable with people, I felt more compassionate toward people. I felt that the fear and the anxiety that this situation created only allowed me to be half of who I am, and so I felt that, because I was so shrouded in fear and self-protection, the MDMA took some of that away. It created this space for who I really am. After that session, I was able to really connect with people and myself in a much better way.

There's a side story here. Before my first MDMA session, my husband, Ben, at the time, sat me down and made a shocking confession. He reminded me that before we got married, I had asked him if he ever had any experiences with men, and did he ever think he was gay? At the time, he said no to both those questions, but this time, he said, "Remember when you asked me those questions? Well, I wasn't completely honest with you. In my past, I have had experiences with men. I'm mildly bisexual, but it's nothing for you to worry about."

For a while, I was really upset, and then I got over it. I thought, he didn't cheat on me; it's in the past; now, we're married. Everything's fine, great. Then, I did the MDMA, and although nothing specifically about my husband came out during the first session, a month later, I was writing in my journal and all of a sudden I got this incredible insight into the situation with my husband. I got a very strong feeling that he had cheated on me. The message was: Your husband cheated on you. He may say that he hasn't, but don't believe a word he says. The MDMA created that access to my inner self, and my inner self very clearly spoke to me, saying, "You've got to listen to this message now. Now that you and I have connected, you need to hear this." The message was: Don't believe a word he says. Confront him, and if he doesn't fess up, you're out of here. You've got to get out.

I confronted him, he denied it, and then a day later, he handed me a letter that basically said, "You're right, I did cheat on you with a man, and I'm so sorry. I wasn't going to tell you, and blah blah blah, but I know that your intuition is very strong, and I wanted to honour that. You're not crazy; you're right."

I know that this information came to me after my first MDMA session, because I was open. The MDMA gave me complete access to my intuition.

We ended up working through the sexuality issues, and I felt that everything was fine. Almost a year later, I did my second MDMA session. He dropped me off at the session, we hugged, and everything was fine. I didn't think that anything about our marriage would come up in the session.

The second session turned out to be the hardest. It killed me, that session. It was crazy. God, I went in thinking I would revisit the Salt Lake City situation, which I could deal with, because it was in the past. But the second session made me deal with the present. My memories of this session are the most vague, especially in the beginning, because the outcome was so powerful. There was not as much anxiety in the beginning, and it was almost peaceful. But then, all of a sudden, I got hit with a brutal truth: "Ben is gay; Ben is gay; Ben is gay." These words were screaming at me. It was incessant. It was a voice that just wouldn't go away.

I remember taking off my eye mask and thinking, "My God, what do I do with this?" I was definitely resisting. I didn't want to deal.

I put the mask back on, and the voice returned, saying, "Okay, you can't handle this information. Clearly, it's too much. I'm screaming at you, because it's so vital, but I'm going to give you something to help you take this back and change your life in the way you need to change your life."

It was a visual, and the visual was of two paths. The first path was my life with Ben, and that life was like a desert, where there was no life. I saw a neon sign flashing the word, "Barren." B-A-R-R-E-N, like an old neon motel sign. Life with Ben was a barren, lifeless desert existence. But then, it showed me the path without Ben, which was the most beautiful visual. I saw a purple colour that I'd never, ever seen in my normal day-to-day life. It was the most beautiful purple colour—the colour of luscious, life-loving, joy and richness. I saw that my life without Ben was rich and full of life, and there was wine, and there were grapes, and there were fruits of all colours. I was very clearly showing myself how beautiful my life would be if I make the brutal decision to leave Ben. The voice very clearly said, "Get out. Go. Leave Ben. Leave Ben. Leave Ben. Leave Ben."

As the MDMA wore off, I felt the worst I've ever felt. I remember the horror of thinking, "Oh, my God, from this moment on, I've crossed the line, and there's no turning back." My attendant said, "Don't make any decisions for six weeks. Just acknowledge that you've got your information, and it's enormous."

I came up with all sorts of rationales for the information I received during that session. I convinced myself that it wasn't actually about leaving Ben. I told myself that it was really to scare the shit out of me, so I can get motivated to work. I was coming up with whatever I could to not have to face reality and make a decision I didn't want to make. But after six weeks had passed, I knew that there was no other way; I had to leave. It was the hardest, most brutal thing I've ever done in my life, but what happened is that my life turned out to be exactly what that visual promised. My life improved vastly after I left Ben. Vastly.

Within a month, I got an incredible work opportunity. Also, I used to be terrified of speaking in public, and all of a sudden, I'm speaking in public. I had none of the social anxiety. It was like the shackles had been taken off me, in every facet. Everything that was horrible transformed into something wonderful. I was soaring.

I remember telling my therapist that I would never trade what I have now to go back. I would never give this up, because this is the richness, love, and beauty of life that I've always been looking for, and the peace that I've been looking for and never accessed, and I wouldn't trade it for anything.

Life was beautiful, but I started to feel that my work still was not done. I'd worked through my issues with Ben, but I still had this unexplained memory from the first session. The full picture from the Salt Lake City incident had not been given to me, and so I was ready to do a third session. Also, there were signs in my life that were showing me that something was ready to be revealed. The first thing that happened to me was when I was washing dishes. I started having a bit of a panic attack, hyper-ventilating, and I thought something sexual happened in that room, and I couldn't access it. Then, I read an essay by another client. I read her piece, and I was in the middle of it, and the paper literally jerked out of my hand. I've never had that kind of physical response before. It jerked out of my hand, and I started hyperventilating and hysterically crying. My inner self said, "Don't read this, you're not ready for this."

Then, I had some sessions with my therapist, where I talked about my extremely painful periods. She said, "You're going through a lot right now. Maybe we should deal with the period pain issue later on." I said, "Why, because I could have been potentially sexually abused?" And when I said that, this wave went through my body, like *joop*, almost like a revelation. I didn't know where I was, and I didn't know what happened. She asked, "What is your body telling you after this wave?" It said to deal with this with kid gloves, that I had to be really gentle on myself.

Then, one day in November, I woke up at my friend's house, and I immediately wrote down, "My friend's father opened the door into the room in the middle of the night and took me into another room and molested me." I just wrote this in my diary. I didn't even have to think; it just came to me. But I didn't really think anything of it.

In January, I did my third session. My third session was, "Yes, the person you suspected molested you, molested you. It wasn't violent; you enjoyed it. You got a lot of attention; this guy was in love with you; this guy was sick. It was in the middle of the night; it happened repeatedly. This is what you've been looking for, and you're now ready to see it." This was the gentlest of sessions I had, even though the revelation was difficult. It was much easier to live with what happened, than it was to suspect something had happened and not knowing what.

It was my friend's father who molested me. He's since passed away. It just made sense. It was like, yes, this happened. Again, it answered so many questions about what I was like as a child. It answered the puzzle piece I was missing, which was, I had known at a very early age—this was when I was four or five years old— that this is what one does when you're alone with an older man.

We were living across the street from this guy. When it came time to go to Salt Lake City, and I was left alone with our family friend, I just assumed that we were going to interact in that same way. I guess he freaked out; why is a four- or five-year-old child trying to do something sexual? This is not right. That's when he attacked me.

And then, he said it's our secret and promised not to tell anyone. I thought, what could an adult possibly have on a four- or five-year-old kid? But he did have something on me! I was trying to engage him sexually as a four- or five-year-old, because that's what I thought one did with an older man.

All of a sudden, I was just like, I have my picture. I know what happened to me, it makes sense. But then, I realised the trauma of this Salt Lake City incident was much more substantial than the trauma of the sexual abuse, because I was being severely punished for something that I didn't know was bad. I've grown up with this idea that I'm the bad one; I'm the naughty one. I thought I was the one that was wrong, not realising that someone taught me this behaviour. I didn't know it was wrong, so this guy just attacked me for being myself. That was much more traumatic, the attack.

I don't know if I've fully come to terms with the sexual abuse yet. I was angry for a while; I was sad, but I was more relieved to have finally gotten the information. Since then, I've had so much energy. All of a sudden, the energy that used to hide this stuff is now freed up for other things. It's almost like I've been deprived of so much joy, excitement, fun, and feeling. Feeling, that's what it is. I've been numbed. I'm over-consuming, because my body is needing all those things to be filled that were empty for so long. So, I think I'm in that phase, and just coming to the end of the phase of gobbling all of life's beauty, because I've denied it to myself for so long—I've been the bad one; I've been the naughty one. Now, I can see that he did this to me. That was not me.

I'm grateful, that's the main thing, for this work. I never would have found out without this work. I know it 100 percent, because I have tried everything. I'm one of those people who grew up in a New Age family; any sort of new technique that was available, from hypnosis to neuro-linguistic programming, to EMDR (Eye Movement Desensitization and Reprocessing), I've done it. Nothing had gotten me even close to what this work has done. It breaks my heart to think of the time, energy, and money one spends to get to find out what's ailing them and not even being close to it. I was so far removed from my own reality.

I suspected Ben was gay a few months after I met him, and I

just thought, no, I must be crazy. There was a voice in my head repeatedly telling me he was gay, but I didn't trust that voice. Now, I'm in touch with that voice. Of course, there's always the paranoid voice, but I know when the true voice comes through and tells me what I need to know, it's true. I now have direct access to my true inner self. Not even direct access, there's no disconnect anymore between who I am on the outside and who I am on the inside. And the MDMA really, really sealed that bond.

The lesson of all this is I will always trust in the medicine and in myself. Always. Because I have so much proof, it's unbelievable. I have so much proof from how I'm in flow. I'm in flow with my life. And I was not for my whole life. I've always been a joyous person, so luckily, I've had that getting me through the hard stuff. I've had wonderful things happen to me. I'm privileged, and I am blessed in so many ways.

Those three sessions are really the most important experiences of my life, hands down. We know that life throws us brutal things, and I always get scared. What's around the corner for me? I'm a waiting-for-the-other-shoe-to-drop kind of person, because of all I've experienced. I've had a lot of bad stuff. But, I just think I'll always be able to handle it, because I have this medicine. I'll always be able to find peace in whatever it is I'm going through, because as long as it's truthful, and the medicine shows me the truth, that's it.

I've become an advocate for the work. I got my whole family involved—my brother, my mom, my dad's partner, and my cousins. That's a lot of family members. And everyone's better for it. Mine was definitely the heaviest compared to everyone else's. I guess that's just my life. So far, it's been a three-year process, a long process. But worth every minute.

The disturbance to Tawny's psyche from the grossly premature sex-ualisation she had suffered cannot be calculated, but it is testimony to her fortitude that she was able to stay focused as the medicine unravelled and made sense of the twists and turns of her abuse. This making sense can be brutal and potentially destabilising, but she has persisted in following the inner truths that have been presented to her in MDMA sessions with journaling, therapy, breathwork and other somatic techniques to establish the truth of the matter. The effect on her career and her outer process has been to bring her to a level of success unachieved before the medicine work. Her focus on integration has been invaluable and sustaining as her inner process continues to unfold.

•   •   •

My chemical imbalance.

Lucy V.

For us to expose ourselves to MDMA, when we are cognitively aware of the trauma and abuse we have suffered as a child, is a singular act of courage. But as Lucy's testimony describes, it was manageable, closer to a revisit than a reliving, and by allowing the medicine to bring her to the core emotional memory of her abuse, her trauma resolved in one session. Witnessing her encounter was to see this mature woman pulling at the flesh on her arms and wringing her hands as she met the terrible events and stayed with them. This is the key, allowing the psyche time to realise that what had happened in the past is not happening in the present. This understanding allows what Ivor Browne calls 'the frozen present', memories known or unknown that we have carried with us willy-nilly throughout our lives, to unfreeze. What had previously been only a remembered memory of her abuse was experienced in-session with the terrible emotions that had remained unfelt, enabling the psyche to release her from their grip.

I am a sixty-year-old woman, married for thirty-one years with one daughter and one stepdaughter and family. My husband

and I are retired and live in a beautiful home near our kids. And I am a victim of sexual abuse, occurring over a period of months when I was a child. I was abused by a beloved family member.

I hadn't told anyone about this part of my childhood, because I thought I had dealt with it. It was over, and the person who violated me had not been emotionally well at the time; I was certain it couldn't be his fault. So, the incidents were safely tucked away in my deepest psyche. I never forgot what had happened; it was not a repressed memory. It was something I chose not to look at and not to talk about. I was a person who did whatever was necessary to make everything all right. In a very large family, including seven children, it's better not to make waves or cause incidents. The less said the better.

However, and realistically, I have been in the business of trying to feel "normal" since the age of about ten. I seemed to feel, and quite often, that something was "missing" in the way I was made up. I was rarely comfortable and was far from feeling normal. Thus, my life became a continuing journey of self-medication (as I now know)—alcohol, drugs, dysfunctional relationships, trying to feel "up," "down," numb, or wild and crazy. My diagnoses have included alcoholism, depression, anxiety, severe eating disorder, bipolar disorder, and on and on. I have taken nearly every antidepressant, anti-psychotic, and anti-anxiety medication available, basically non-stop and overlapping since I was twenty-one-years old. The long-running thought was that I suffered from "clinical depression," something biological that I was to live with the rest of my life—a chemical imbalance. I would never really feel "great" again, but would have to live with just getting by 'white-knuckling' through life.

Then, at some point in my forties, I did tell a psychiatrist about the abuse. Long story short: It was now part of my file, but was never really addressed by anyone again.

I did have times in my life when I was better; those times were usually the result of my environment. For instance, when I had my daughter, or visiting my family, getting married, landing a new job. But inevitably, those feelings of joy ended, and for what reason, I didn't know. Everyone just concurred that my "clinical depression" was the culprit, my "chemical imbalance."

I was aware of many drugs, as I was either prescribed them or self-medicated for mood-altering purposes. I did not know that some of the so-labelled 'bad' ones or 'illegal' ones were used in progressive therapies until my twenty-three-year-old daughter, who had been following research and studies, suggested I try a drug therapy used for PTSD. The medicine would be MDMA. I simply trusted her and agreed to meet with an attendant familiar with the process. My daughter and I agreed that it couldn't make things worse.

The day of my session, I was introduced to a very comfortable atmosphere, and I was not afraid, just curious. The attendant agreed to be with me and help me use this medicine to its most beneficial potential.

First, I shared with him as much as I could about my abuse. It was not something I could verbalise, and yet, it was important, because I needed to focus on an intention before beginning the process. I needed to draw the connection between the abuse and my life since. It was becoming clear that I had a huge disconnect, and yet, had no idea how to fix it. This was my goal going into the session.

As the medicine took effect, I became comfortable. It was quite a pleasant feeling, and my guide told me to simply stay with it. I wasn't required to do or say anything. But I wanted to return to my goal; I needed to talk. The medicine relieved me of any anxiety and allowed me not to relive the experiences of my abuse, but rather to revisit them, take a look, talk about it in detail (which I had NEVER been able to do previously), and decide that I could live with it as part of my life. But I knew almost immediately and through discussion afterward, those incidences of abuse had lost their power to control.

For the very first time that I could remember, I felt as though it would all be okay, and that I didn't have to work so hard at living every day. I went back to my life, and I felt good! I didn't understand exactly what was different, but it was. I still have struggles and challenges, bad days. But I used to wake nearly every day, wondering how I could make it through the next twenty-four hours; I haven't felt that way since before my medicine session.

A couple of months after the session, I went to visit my brother who had suffered a stroke. The thought of that visit brought some kind of terror to me. Making the plans and the drive there was pure anxiety. Where was that comforting feeling I had somewhere in me after the medicine therapy? I lost it, I thought, or maybe it didn't exist at all.

My brother's wife can be a very controlling, bitter, and angry person (for a lot of good reasons) who requires one to choose each and every word meticulously so as not to upset her. I had always been afraid of speaking to her; I didn't want to anger or hurt her. Not even a phone call. After a tense eight-hour drive, I walked into their home. And then, it happened so vividly and stunningly, I was shocked.

My fear dissolved in my body. I had no fear of her or the situation. I felt bad for her, but I was totally okay. And it lasted throughout my visit. And it lasted when I came home. And it lasts to this day.

I now know, because of my abuse when I was young, that I simply lived in fear of people, situations, future and past, myself, people I knew and didn't know. And I really don't understand why, and I don't really need to know why today. In the past, I felt isolated and different. I felt "less than." Today, I feel connected to the human race, people I know and don't know. I feel a spiritual connection to all people, and that I belong.

I had not told anyone in my family about my session with MDMA. I was sure I would get disapproval, which right now, I don't care much about. But it just wasn't necessary for me to share. However, my sister, who was on that visit to my brother with me, asked me what was different. She said she had never seen me so "settled." Was it a new medication that finally works? New psychiatrist? No. I shared my story with her, a person who had never had an illegal drug or even been drunk. After much discussion, she is now a convert to the idea and feels, as do I, that this therapy needs to be made available for all individuals suffering with PTSD.

I think quite often about how I can express this epiphany which came to my life. I am reminded of the old "magic eye" pictures. Just pages of what looked like wallpaper samples. They said, "You'll see a Bengal tiger in that picture." I searched and searched.

Yes, well maybe there or there, but then, not really. Then someone suggested, "Don't look so hard, relax your eyes." And what appeared was a huge Bengal tiger that I will forever see in that picture. It will be there as long as I give up searching so desperately and allow it to appear. Just as my experience with MDMA. I've been to a place that will forever be there. I can draw from that as I need.

I still have situations and times that are challenging. I get upset with myself and often don't understand my choices or conditions. However, it usually just takes a moment of my realisation that, "I'll be okay, I am okay," for me to instantly be in a better place. I am, very simply, free from the paralysing fear that ruled my life. And I credit my very wise and intuitive daughter, MDMA therapy, the medicine, and the attendant, for this very amazing reconnection to life.

Lucy has deservedly been restored to normal function in her life, and nine years after her session she is thriving; "I'm doing really wonderfully," she says today. Her gratitude for the healing she achieved is immense, saying, "My only regret is that I didn't find this medicine when I was much younger; that should be a goal of ours. I did a lot of unnecessary damage over all those years." With her daughter who introduced her to the work, Lucy advocates energetically for the healing potential of this remarkable medicine to become known and available to people who need it, people who know everything about its reputation as a 'party drug' but absolutely nothing about its healing potential.

But with robust support and the love of her family, Lucy has come to a very different place in her life. Her joyous life force, previously compromised by her inner confusion, is restored. Her gratitude to the

*work for enabling this revelation is boundless; the truth, presented
in all its horror, has set her free.*

● ● ●

This is, of course, a process, and it seems to continue without end.

Anne

Anne is a PhD psychologist whose work with MDMA began as a result of supporting her daughter, H., who was starting to do the work. She had come in solidarity to sit with the attendant as she sat with H., and seeing the outcomes in her daughter, decided to do the work herself. In Anne's own sessions, the favour would be returned, and H. and the attendant would sit with her. Anne was spiritually extremely aware and very sensitive to the medicine, taking to it like a duck to water. Over multiple sessions, she enjoyed revelation after revelation with complete surrender and a fierce focus. With one exception, she only ever took the first dose of 125 mg.

There is nothing to be afraid of anymore
I have already spent all my fear
trying to take care of young infants
and toddlers and small children
my own deep inside me
Nothing ever goes anywhere

Unresolved trauma roots in the body
finds a spot in the bone, the sinew the organ
and then sends out tendrils
wherever it can find the space
often showing up where we lease expect it
not recognising it for what it is
And yet it is never too late to have a happy childhood
because that never goes anywhere either
all the possibilities and potential
that we bring in when we incarnate
that is here too

I was diagnosed with Parkinson's Disease several years ago. My own sense of my movement disorder was that it was the result of the trauma I had experienced as an infant and small child. I had heard that MDMA was being used successfully to treat trauma and decided to try it. I was sixty-five-years old and had no previous history with drugs of any kind. I did a series of twenty sessions over a period of one-and-a-half years.

MDMA brought me back to life. My first session was the happiest and the most exciting experience I'd ever had in this lifetime. I knew myself outside of the strain of trauma for the first time, and it was glorious. I kept saying, "This is life? I can do this!" I felt so safe and so happy and grateful to have finally found this place in myself. I knew that I was both a blessing and being blessed, and that there was no need to 'figure things out' but simply to let my being effortlessly unwind and unfold to its true nature.

This medicine has gifted me along three paths: The personal, the interpersonal, and the transpersonal. In the personal realm, it allowed me to see my life with such clarity and compassion. I have been able to access infant and toddler trauma in a rare and deeply useful way. I see the trauma and understand its impact on my life and development. I see my weaknesses and woundings and understand their impact on loved ones without judgement or guilt but simply able to see things as they are. I can see my parents and caregivers with compassion and understand who they were, and what they were struggling with as they raised me. More significantly, MDMA has enabled me to actually change deep patterns and change how I perceive the world and myself. This is, of course, a process, and it seems to continue without end.

In the interpersonal realm, MDMA helped me to unwind personal knots that were longstanding and deep with my beloved daughter. The MDMA that we were both doing simply opened us up to one another in a way that was beautiful and profound. It let the love that had always been there become more clear and true. Our children absorb our unresolved material so easily, and I am so very grateful to have had the chance to scrub some of that clean and make room for new ways of being to emerge between us.

The biggest surprise for me with MDMA has been in the transpersonal realm. From the first session on, I fully embodied what I call the shamanic/priest realm. I found myself chanting in languages I do not know and gesturing with great authority in gestures I do not know. It felt like performance art for the soul as the shamans worked to heal the baby, with me playing all the parts. The first time, it was quite confusing to me. What was this? Who am I? Over time, I came to see that this shamanic material is simply an expression of more than I am and has come into play to serve my greater healing. Connecting with this aspect of my being has allowed me to meet parts of myself I deeply love and explains much of what I have been drawn to in this lifetime.

MDMA seems to quiet the habitual part of my brain, so I can experience myself and the world outside of my normal patterns of perception. Better than any spiritual practice I have found, it momentarily dismantles the grip of the ego and shows me the truer song that I sing. It opens the gate for the river of God to flow freely, and then I must find my way to bridge what it has shown me and my current configuration of self. I remain eternally grateful for the opportunity to have met this compound and learn from the wisdom and beauty within myself that it has shown me.

Dissemble yourselves
we are not fixed
but fluid
We hold ourselves
in postures and shapes
believing we are that
but we are not
We are burning water
lit with love

Anne's observation about how children 'absorb our unresolved material so easily' comports with a profound statement by Carl Jung, "The greatest influence on the life of the child is the unlived life of the parents." We can only act from what we know, doing the best we can with the information available to us. Only when we can finally learn the truth about what really happened to us do we become able to act from this place of greater self-knowledge. The recalibration of the relationship between Anne and her daughter has been profound, enabling them to 'unwind personal knots' from the considerable traumas in both their lives. Her Parkinson's continues, but she writes, "I am doing remarkably well and have very few symptoms these days."

•   •   •

I knew I was searching to get to something deeper.

N. S-J.

N's testimony in this book speaks to the ability of MDMA to reveal to us the darkest events of our childhood, often one-by-one, and her session-work echoes this action. From shadowy intimations floating around when she was suicidal, the medicine has shown her the horror of events in her upbringing and released her from the worst of her dysfunction. In every session, new memories emerge, many of which have been corroborated by family members, and her task post-session is to reenter her life with resolve to integrate the information as best she can. Bravely.

What led me to pursue MDMA? I started dating this guy, and I was falling in love with him. I had only been in a romantic, long-term relationship with a woman in college in Botswana, and that was the first time in a long span that I didn't feel suicidal.

I had never fallen in love with any man at that point in my life, and I really felt I was losing my mind, like very flared attachment issues. I thought I had a solid sense of self-worth; I like myself and love myself, but it punctured a wound that was like a blind spot that I didn't even really know was there.

I had been depressed and had thoughts of suicide my whole life. That was just part of who I was, and I'm very open and loving, too. Being with him, when he would want space, or we would have a fight, I felt I was disintegrating and didn't know who I was anymore. It was very scary. I know our relationship made certain things flare up for him too. It made us look at things we needed to look at about ourselves.

But it was hard, really ugly. We would get together and break up, on and off again and again. I felt like if I was not with this guy, I was going to die. I was acting irrationally, with fits of rage. I was alarmed at myself, and he was too. Friends I was talking to were concerned.

I met my MDMA attendant at a women's full moon gathering. I had gotten her information for my partner, because I knew that he had attachment issues with his mother. I thought that this work would benefit him. Maybe three months later, he got in touch with the attendant and had a session. He said it was incredible. That same week, I had had a major upset. I was really depressed and anxious, feeling suicidal, not knowing what was even going on with me, just very confused.

I had been in talk therapy since I was about thirteen, because I was cutting myself for about two years, on and off. At a certain point, my mother, a therapist, found out. I imagine I wanted her to. She sent me to therapy. That was definitely helpful. I was seeing a psychiatrist doing talk therapy. She was always an advocate of putting me on medication, and so was my mother. My gut always told me that was not going to be the answer. I was clear on that.

I was on Ritalin in high school for focus, and I guess depression too. I didn't like it. Then, in college, I was on Vyvanse and Adderall. They helped me focus but ultimately made me a bit moody. Then, at some point in college, I was on an antidepressant for a month. I said, "I don't want to continue this." I knew I was searching to get to something deeper.

I had always said a mantra, like, "Oh, I have a chemical imbalance." That's what I had been told by my psychiatrist. That seemed to be the only thing that might make sense, so I stuck with that. But I was always searching for deeper things. When I first heard about MDMA (I had tried ecstasy, or Molly, before), I was thinking about my partner. I told my attendant, "He is detached from his emotions. He's a sociopath." He's nowhere near a sociopath, but he does have trouble accessing emotions.

He came back just raving about how it was such an incredible experience. He advocated for me doing it. He had this blissful experience. He said he saw all the chakras align, and they were so powerful. I really wanted to do the work, but I was scared. I was like, "Stuff's going to come up."

I had a major upset. I was crying non-stop, panicked that he wanted to leave me, which he probably did, and I wanted to leave. It was just such a mess. I ended up leaving his place and going to a friend's nearby. I took a taxi there, just to get there immediately and try to calm down. I texted my attendant that night, and we scheduled a talk in the morning. I said, "Look, I'm losing it. I need help."

I had called my mom, too, that night, just sobbing. Her thing, when I'm clearly not doing well, is always like, "Well, you might want to call the doctor and get on a medication." It's the last thing I want to hear. Did hold it in my mind, though. If it's this bad, you know what? Maybe that's an option. I needed to do something. Things were not working out.

At the time, I was living in my grandmother's apartment. It's vacant, so I was staying there after college. I had lived there with a roommate for a year, and then alone for six or eight months. When I was with the roommate, I told her, "I think there's a ghost in this house." I kept saying that. I would tell friends that would come over, too. Everyone was just like, "Oh, ha, ha! Like, maybe, yeah." I would laugh, too, because it seemed weird, but I was very clear that something was up with that house.

I practice Buddhist chanting, *nam myoho renge kyo*. When I would chant at my altar with this mandala, the *gohonzon*, I would feel like someone was walking up behind me every now and then. Sometimes, I would see my grandmother's husband. That morning, before I left the house to go work with my attendant, I chanted, and I saw his demon face. It's like somehow, my body knew that was going to surface.

I was nervous, but not super scared. I felt good about it. I think of myself as brave, and I'm going to do what I'm going to do. I told someone, "I'm going to battle for myself when I do this work."

I went in thinking I was going to work through stuff with my dad, because he is an alcoholic, has been for all my life, and he has rage issues. My parents weren't together; when I would see him, sometimes, he would seemingly ignore me. That was always tough. I had a lot of anger toward him that I had never fully expressed, so I thought I was going to work on that or work through that. But nothing with him came up.

Before I took the first dose, I expressed a concern that when I had taken Molly recreationally, sometimes, it was wonderful, totally joyous, but a couple of times, I had an experience where I got really depressed before I got high, or just really depressed and then never got high. Both of those things have happened. I was worried that it would be something like that. That first time with MDMA I did get depressed for a second. It was just terror and then it went away. I told my attendant, and she said, "Oh, well, just relax," and then it went away.

She was playing music, just relaxing, classical music, but I requested jazz. I asked her to put on Miles Davis, because my dad was always playing jazz growing up. I thought that would help me get back into what it was like being with him in his house. She put Miles Davis on, and then I just, very soon after, felt like a child in my dad's house, listening to Miles Davis. But I didn't spend much time there.

It was almost like watching a movie. I'm a filmmaker, so I'm just intrigued by how it feels; you're watching a movie, but a movie that you're in. It's weird, because it's just one moment, but it seemed to stretch on for so long. I saw myself in my grandmother's apartment (where I was living at the time), in my grandmother's bedroom with my step-grandfather, and he was fingering me very violently. I saw it like a cartoon. He was just sort of flush red and so cartoony. I remember him and being in pain. Then, physically, I was in the fetal position, blocking my vagina and just wincing in pain, seemingly for hours of the session.

Other instances of abuse have come to the surface for me at different points since the session, through dreams, in waking life; walking around or at work, I'll just have a vision of something.

Before this, I had no idea that this had happened to me. None. I tried to explain to my family and to have it make sense to them, because I know it just didn't make sense to them. Some of the other memories that surfaced, they weave into things that I knew, that weren't suppressed. That's what really solidifies it. It's all just woven stuff, or like a puzzle. After, I remember dancing in the mirror for my grandfather. I would dance, and he would watch me. In the session, it's definitely work. It was difficult. When you're doing this work and you take the MDMA, it doesn't feel like there's any decision to go to any area. It just takes you. After, I was totally in shock. I walked and walked for miles. It was nice. It felt good.

I knew I had found the root. There was no question. That felt like a relief. I felt like I wasn't crazy for the first time in my life, which was incredible. I always thought I was going to struggle with depression my whole life. I was like, "Oh, you know, sure, I'll be happy sometimes, but I don't know, this is always going to be a problem." Now that it's something that I'm working on and working through, I feel like I have my life back.

That's why this work is so insanely powerful. I think of so many people and how traumatised we are, and how rampant sexual abuse is, and violence, and how it affects us, and how it can have a grip on you for your entire life. This is a way to look at it and let it go. You can actually do that.

This work really allows you to look at yourself with compassion and kindness. You were hurt in a way that's hideous, but there's a way out of this. The worst, most horrific things, people can overcome with this work.

Since the session, I think I have a better sense of boundaries. I'm a pretty transparent person. Boundaries have been hard for me. In the second session, a lot of stuff with my mom came up, that my step-grandfather was abusing me and her; she knew he was abusing me and just this whole web. She is in complete denial, though. She just says none of it happened. She pretty much raised me on her own, and we always had a difficult relationship, but also very close, almost too close, like super enmeshed. As I have grown up, I've worked to have boundaries with her. I feel more clarity around that.

I still get depressed, which is a struggle. But now, I feel like it's something I'm working on, and not like I'm always going to be this way. I've done two sessions. I'm hoping to have another one in maybe a month or two. So, it makes sense that I'm still working through all of it.

The abuse that came up in the second session was so deep. I'm still processing it. Years ago, I had asked my mom about when she saw clients as a psychologist, what that was like, and she had mentioned something about someone raping a baby. It was just like, "You know, I had a lot of hard cases. This was one of them." It struck me as very weird, because that was the only thing she'd ever said about her work. I thought, "Why would I only know that one piece of information? Why is that the only thing you're sharing?"

Then, in my therapist's office, there was a photo of a woman washing, cradling a baby, beautiful photo. And it made me angry. Then, I had a dream. Something in the dream told me I had been abused as a baby. I was like, "That's really far out. Maybe it's true. Maybe it's not." In the session, it came up that he had raped me as an infant.

I knew I was a baby, and there was just this evil energy. I knew he was inside me. I don't really have the words, because I didn't have the words then, I guess. Then, I remember seeing my mom. Somehow, she knew. I don't know how, but she was just sobbing, just distraught, just totally.

He was abusing her, too, which came up for me when I did the medicine work. I remembered he would come into the house at night and rape me. I thought, "Oh, maybe he just left after," but then in the session, what came up was I'm sitting in my room, and he is in there with her, and she's just crying and screaming. That offered a little bit more compassion for her.

I told my dad about the first session. He kept saying, "If this really did happen," and all that sort of language, so I stopped talking about it with him. When I was going to have the second session, I told him. At first, he was resistant, and then, he agreed. I've told my mom everything. I told my aunt most of this stuff, not the infant stuff. It's too much. Even the other day, I talked to my aunt on the phone, and we were kind of hashing it out. It wasn't nasty, but it wasn't nice. She's a lawyer, so she was arguing as to why this couldn't have happened, which is so infuriating.

I asked her, because I'm trying to get more of a timeframe for everything and still piecing things together. My grandmother and my step-grandfather started dating when my aunt was fifteen, and my mom was in college. So, now I'm thinking, maybe he abused my aunt, too. I asked her what she remembers about him, and she just said, "He was fine. He was nice." She didn't say much, and Mom doesn't say much. I think that's a signifier of having blocked the person out. Because if anyone had asked me about him, before the therapy, I would've said that he was creepy and quiet, but I can't tell you much about him. I feel like they can't, either.

My aunt said she's consulted doctor friends of hers. She claims that people have said that this can induce memories that aren't real. I don't know if there's data out there that says that. It doesn't make any sense to me. You don't make this stuff up. Also, I had experiences where certain things came up later, that I discovered in-session. In my first session, I had half a story about my dad's friend who kind of was violent toward me, and my dad's friend later confirmed it. My dad thought I was crazy, and then he called his friend, and his friend told the identical story, minus a couple of details. This was a memory I had no memory of until I had the session.

The person that sexually abused me died. My dad's friend who was violent toward me, after I got the story corroborated, I just decided I don't want to deal. I'm not going to need to contact him. I was looking for a place to live after this came up. I said, "I cannot live with my mom." I don't make enough money to pay rent in the city. I asked my boyfriend if I could move in. He felt pressured, because it came up in panic, like, "I don't make enough money to pay rent, and I can't live with my mom, so, I need to live here. If I can't live here, you don't actually care about me." It did not go well, having the conversation be raised in that way. But since then, I've looked for a place. It's hard, searching for a place.

So, for the past two months, I've been staying with him. It's funny, because he had a lot of reservations about living together, but we have a great time. I don't know. We're still talking about me transitioning to be with my mom a few days a week, or a couple of days a week, which I do not want to do. At first, I was looking at it as like a death sentence. I could barely even go there. I don't see it as a death sentence anymore, but it's still hard.

N's work has continued with more revelations about the severe abuse she suffered as a child and infant. Her recovery from this horror is a work-in-progress, but she has found that the truth of her childhood, disgusting as it was, has liberated her from a pernicious idea. The quick-and-easy diagnosis made by her psychiatrist was there was something congenitally wrong with her; she had a chemical imbalance. Thanks, doc. The only thing wrong with this young woman is she was consistently and foully sexually abused by family members and others from infancy. For 'professionals,' trick-cyclists of the first order, to inflict their wilful ignorance upon her in the form of a completely false diagnosis and make her dependent on prescription drugs that only numb her pain (and every other feeling) is to atomise the Hippocratic Oath, "First, Do No Harm." Every single system within her, from her brain circuitry to her ability to develop mentally and achieve normal sexual maturity as she became a woman, was understandably and terribly compromised, resulting in the 'flared' issues she encountered when she first fell in love. Chemical imbalance; really?

CHAPTER TWO

Changing the Perception

———

"I know that most men, including those at ease with problems of the greatest complexity, can seldom accept even the simplest and most obvious truth if it be such as would oblige them to admit the falsity of conclusions which they have delighted in explaining to colleagues, which they have proudly taught to others, and which they have woven, thread by thread, into the fabric of their lives."

LEO TOLSTOY

REGRETTABLE REPUTATION

With all that this medicine can accomplish with responsible use, it is extremely unfortunate its reputation has become so tarnished. MDMA is both trivialised and demonised, seen as a party drug for young people who just want to have fun but who, by taking an impure version from the street, may also suffer consequences requiring medical attention, making the medicine appear to be of concern.

To many people, it doesn't seem credible that MDMA could possibly also have a role as a medicine and have passed on the opportunity.

NEW PERSPECTIVE

When trauma overpowers us to the point that our organism is overwhelmed, the hypervigilant psyche moves decisively to override the fear by putting us into a non-ordinary state of consciousness. In that condition, the psyche captures the emotional and cognitive memory of the traumatic event to protect us from the full realisation of what has occurred. The way our traumatic memories become captured, unknowable to our conscious awareness, occurs in an instant, absent our volition or knowledge. We are helpless victims, and it is done to us, for our benefit, by the protective psyche. Something quite beyond ordinary consciousness happens to us in response to a life-threatening situation, enabling us to become separated, or dissociated, from the trauma.

To release these memories from their captured state, we need to return to a non-ordinary state of our own volition, so the psyche can understand that now is not then. MDMA allows us the perfect opportunity to do that.

It is beyond the scope of this book to describe in detail the complex mechanism-of-action of MDMA. What we offer here is an overview.

Our brains are constantly required to maintain a basic level of serotonin for mood stabilisation, enabling our emotional balance. The action of MDMA produces copious amounts of serotonin for a few hours, flooding the brain to produce the familiar feeling of extreme well-being that characterises its use. Work with this medicine takes advantage of the non-ordinary state of consciousness resulting from this radical but temporary increase of serotonin levels in the brain.

MDMA increases the quantity of serotonin released into the synapse by stimulating a massive release of stored serotonin from vesicles in the pre-synaptic membrane. This action floods the synaptic gap and leads to significant increases in serotonin becoming available in the synapse. Additionally, re-uptake inhibition blocks the recycling of serotonin that would normally draw it away from the synapse back into the releasing cell. Operationally, oxytocin release also creates feelings of trust, bonding, and openness. Dopamine release accounts for the energised, focused feelings and a desire to talk.

Interested readers will find the mechanism-of-action of MDMA described in considerable detail in Chapter Four of the book, *Ecstasy: The Complete Guide*, edited by Julie Holland, M. D.

FROM 5-HTP TO 5-HT

Amino acids are the building blocks of the protein that constitutes 20 percent of our body weight. They are involved in all biological processes, including regulating mood balance in the brain through conversion to serotonin. The chemical name of serotonin is 5-HT, and one amino acid, 5-HTP, is its precursor. Many amino acids require multiple chemical changes to become 5-HT, but the precursor 5-HTP requires only one, making it a particularly valuable ally in this work.

Serotonin is present in our bowels and blood platelets, transmitting impulses between nerve cells and regulating cyclic body processes. It is also present in our brains always, maintaining mood balance and contributing to feelings of well-being. It follows that a plentiful supply of amino acids is essential, if the body is going to be able to produce sufficient 5-HT to maintain emotional balance at acceptable levels.

The action of MDMA upon entering the body is to convert all available amino acids to serotonin. It is very, very efficient at this task and over-produces serotonin to temporarily flood the brain and reliably cause the euphoric sensations associated with MDMA. We use the medicine in doses varying from 75 mg to a maximum of 200 mg, per the client's needs and wishes. When the most commonly requested dose, 125 mg + 75 mg to the 200 mg maximum, is used up in the session, it may be assumed that the supplies of amino acids have been compromised and may also be used up. This leads, immediately after the session, to a temporary depletion of serotonin in the brain, a condition which, if not remedied, can lead to mood destabilisation and depression.

We recommend to our clients they supplement with 100 mg of 5-HTP a few hours after their session has concluded, and morning and night for three days following. Along with good nutrition, this gives the body the raw materials it needs to readily make serotonin to rebalance the levels in the brain, forestalling the possibility of a radical downward mood swing. This strategy has been employed with every client, and though a few have reported feeling "flat" or "unfocused" for a few days following the medicine work, we have had no reports close to clinical depression.

It is also interesting to realise that what is causing the euphoria is not the medicine itself, MDMA, but serotonin, a naturally occurring endogenous substance experienced at high levels.

The split-dose protocol we use was developed by practitioners in the field during the early years of this century and was utilised by Dr. Michael Mithoefer and colleagues throughout their 2010 study, performed under rigorous US government supervision. People familiar with the action of medicine suggested two doses administered over sixty to ninety minutes, one 125 mg followed later by 75 mg, allowed the participant a gentler entry and exit when compared to the full 200 mg dose being administered at one time. Each step is taken in agreement with the client, who has the opportunity to experience how they are feeling in the moment and decide if they want to continue with the complete dose.

In addition to providing a gentle introduction to the medicine, the split-dose protocol extends the effective life of the experience of MDMA. A given dose of MDMA remains active in the body for about four hours. It is consistent. By giving a second dose ninety minutes or so into a session, you extend the session to a five- or six-hour experience. Splitting the doses not only softens the impact of the beginning of the session and makes the ramp-down at the end of the session slow and gentle, it extends the useful active hours of the session.

You're just suddenly dropped into it.

Jennifer J.

Jennifer is a seeker, actively exploring aspects of spirituality and writing on questions of personal belief. As we move along this elevated spectrum, we will undoubtedly encounter any dark and problematic material still residing within us, and her intimation that 'something had happened' turned out to be correct. The full awareness she experienced clarified not only the trauma itself but, significantly, how her beloved parents had somehow been implicated with the event in her mind. With the clarity she experienced, she was able to understand that their role was completely innocent, victims along with their young daughter of the perpetrator's abuse.

It was a friend who helped me out. She brought me to the work. She and I had both been exploring questions around spirituality, and what more is there out there and that sort of thing. She had told me that she had done this work in the past, and that she had been living by it and had seen some good results. As we talked about it, it just was something I was curious about, something I had, at forty-four, never done even recreationally.

I have never used illegal substances or drugs, except I smoked pot probably six times in my life. I had a very, very limited experience with any type of recreational drug. That part of it was a bit scary to me. The idea that it could help release some sort of traumas or anything like that was really intriguing. I had the feeling that having done years and years of traditional talk therapy, starting post 9/11, there was clearly something that had happened when I was younger that was traumatic, that I hadn't released, and I didn't have access to in my conscious mind.

I didn't feel that talk therapy was going to get me there, because I'd done everything I could with that. I do think that was critical work before coming to something like this, because I don't think I would have had the wherewithal to process everything that was going on and handle it and manage it, had I not had all those years of traditional experience.

I had a strong inclination that something had happened, but could not get to it in my rational, talking brain. That had always niggled at me, and I had stopped traditional therapy a few years ago, not in a good or bad way. It just felt like I had come to the end of the line with it. It felt good and stable, and everything was fine.

What brought me to it was a feeling that there was some sort of trauma. I didn't know what it was and didn't know how to access it. I thought that I was at the point in my life where I was ready to deal with it. I thought this would be a way to deal with it.

I would say the first session was fruitful. I was sort of shocked by it, but I had no idea what to expect. The first session was powerful, because, again, I had never done any kind of work like that before. I had no idea what to expect. I was chatty; I was kind of all over the place. I was definitely very outward and chatting and sort of giggling, but it really brought a lot of peace for a lot of things that were happening in my life or had happened in my life. I released a lot of trauma that I was so shocked by, because the first things that came up were my miscarriages. I had two, possibly three miscarriages prior to having my daughter. I was so shocked, because rationally, I knew that those had happened, and I thought I had forgiven myself.

I didn't realise how deep those still were and how much I blamed myself for it. I was really surprised afterward about how much grieving I did during the process, during the session, and got it out of my body. It was kind of incredible. That was the big, profound thing that shifted for me in that session. I think just having that come up and feeling that big shift drew me back to it. I know there is something powerful in this that's worth exploring. I think it will help me get there, because that was something I would never have expected at all, rationally.

I really thought I had worked through it, and I have a healthy child now, was secure in my marriage, and all that was great. I was surprised that came up in the way that it did and how lost or how buried that trauma really was, and how much I blamed myself for it. Then, it just sort of released. That release of it was so profound that I wanted to try this again.

I was kind of coming to thinking: There's this trauma, I'm pretty sure something happened at some point when I was a kid, but I have literally, absolutely no idea what it could be. It didn't come up at all, and what came up was my miscarriages. That was such a raw trauma, because I blamed myself so much for the miscarriages, in a way that in my conscious mind, I definitely did not. Consciously, I knew it wasn't my fault, and I consciously knew I couldn't have done anything different than what I did. It may be over, and I thought I had forgiven whatever. I was really shocked by how much that came up. It really felt like it had moved out of my body during that process.

I usually feel like I have to verbally process things. I'm chatty; I'm a writer now; I process things through words. In that first session, because I didn't really know what I was getting into, even though I had been told, I was chatting, wanting to write stuff down. I was really external in the way I lined up for a session.

I was giggling and talking in a cartoon voice. I was all over the place. It was fun for me. I thought the experience was really good for me, because I felt like what a joyful person I was and how happy I was with my husband and my daughter. I love them, and I was articulating all that in a pure, joyful way. It was reassuring and sort of just humbling in a nice way.

The experience of going through the miscarriage stuff was cathartic. I wasn't reliving it. It was more I was crying and grieving, letting my body grieve in a way that I never had, because I didn't allow myself to when the trauma happened. The response that you're expected to have is to hold it together and be grateful that you got pregnant and that you'll be able to try again. People say, "How soon can you try again? You're good; you can get pregnant," that kind of stuff. That's how you're expected to handle it.

It's supposed to be this private trauma, where it happens early, and nobody knew you were pregnant in the first place, and nobody knows that you lost a pregnancy. Now, being able to cry, I couldn't stop the crying; it just came out. Then, suddenly, it was just done, and I sort of moved on to the next phase.

I did three or four sessions. I think I probably was doing it too close together. I had maybe too much expectation, because I think I was so excited by what happened the first time. I wanted just to get there; I want to get there. I want to get it done. I'm the kind of person who is not going to sit and wallow in self-pity. I'll do that for a minute, and by minute three, it's like I started working on it two minutes ago. I just felt like there was something there, and I could fix it. It was really exciting to me. I was like, "I'm going to try it again, and I will do it again." I did it maybe three months later, and I don't remember what happened in that one, but I felt like I didn't really get anything out of it. It was kind of like, "Use your voice." Looking back, it was quite profound. It took us searching for meaning in all this stuff. I wanted that big revelation again and that didn't happen.

Then, I did it again; I was trying to clear trauma of whatever plus ickiness from my last job. Just trying to clear trauma, whatever had happened in the last few months, almost like a tune-up. I'm sure it was doing something, but I think I was looking for too much meaning in it. I feel like even though that was the last session that we did, I wasn't getting there. I was getting kind of frustrated, and again, I think it's just because I wasn't ready or it wasn't enough time to doing the work in between. It wasn't coming.

Then, I switched to another attendant and requested a different dose, and frankly, I think that's what did it. I think I was probably ready. I had been hitting a wall with what I was doing. Also, I think the atmosphere was more comfortable for me too, because it was easier to get to. It was a quick cab ride home. The place was inviting and room-like, where I didn't feel like I was doing something wrong. I think part of the other reason that I had such good results in the first session was because I did it at home, so I was really enveloped and safe in my space.

In the first sessions, I think I felt that my words were important. I needed to write it down; I had to remember the story. I had to remember the details, like that was the point of it, because that's what therapy is, all the stories. If you don't repeat it to someone, then what happened? What's the point of it? How do you explain what happened, and what the result was? You have to be able to repeat it. That's what I was holding onto. My second sitter got me to stop, saying, "Look, I'll write stuff down, so maybe just be quiet." Then, I don't think I spoke basically the entire time, and that's when I unlocked and it completely changed things.

The big revelation I had in that last one, and the only thing I really remember from the last session, was that note that kept going in my head again and again. It was like, "Who are you without your stories? Oh, then you're free." That's what my mind kept repeating to me. Then, it was like whatever was happening the rest of the session, I don't remember. I don't remember the stories. I went past the story, let myself go deeper. I still think there's more deep places for me to go.

I think I'm so caught up in the stories, because our stories define us. I am so defined by my stories; otherwise, who am I? That's just scary, in your conscious mind; that's a very scary road to go down. I want to hold onto those stories, because they somehow define me.

There's something about letting that go. Even though I don't remember any stories, and I have no narrative to play, there was another trauma that I experienced. There was this other thing over there. I have no idea what. I knew something was happening; bubbles were popping. It was like I was being wrung out, and I can't explain it.

I think if that had happened in the first session, I wouldn't have gone back. I think I needed those Aha's; I needed those revelations; I needed something to hold onto, to justify going back repeatedly. I don't think I would have trusted it if it was just like, "Oh, out of it for a few hours."

In the first session with the second attendant, the trauma just unlocked. It wasn't even like a big, scandalous trauma, but it kind of was, I guess. It was just after I settled into the idea that I was safe. "Just remember that you're safe. Think about if there's any other fear that you might not be addressing, or that you're not looking at, that's blocking you from getting at it and just deal with that."

I guess that slowed me down, and I suddenly really believed that I was safe. Then, the thought switched to, "My daughter is safe. I know she's safe, because I'm her mother. Of course, she's safe." I kept repeating that, and then there was something that clicked. I think it really settled into me. I know she's safe. Then, suddenly the memory just came.

It was just, "Oh, right." It was just like a light went on. It wasn't like I relived it; it wasn't like the whole story played out in front of me; it was just like, "Oh, wait, that's what happened." Like all of a sudden you remembered where you parked, that's what it felt like. Oh, right, the car's on the corner of Walnut and Vine. Suddenly, you remember; you don't have to think about it. You're not like, "Oh, where did I park when I was driving down the road?" It's not the whole thing; it was just, "Oh, shit, of course, I'm parked next to the green box."

Then, it turned into a deep forgiveness for my parents and then understanding why it would have happened. Why would they have let me be in that situation? By understanding the whole *mis-en-scene*, I know it's fine. It was just done. I harbour no anger toward them; I'm totally fine.

As Jennifer allowed the medicine to unfold and reveal the seed kernel of her trauma, she asked out loud, "Could I be making this up?" She's inquisitive, so I asked, "What's the motive?" But answer came there none. That someone would wilfully invent such an event is, of course, possible; but is it likely? And is it likely enough to justify a movement of recovered-memory deniers? Observations from this work and from the many testimonies in this book speak otherwise.

Once the details of the abuse were revealed to her, Jennifer's session turned into forgiveness for her innocent parents and full understanding how they were deceived, of why they would have let her be in the situation that led to her abuse in a 'private audience' with the spiritual leader to whom they had introduced their young daughter.

• • •

What if I were the perpetrator?
Bea A.

Bea had come to the work at the suggestion of her brother. She had been the victim of serial sexual abuse as a young girl, and her family had acted with the only strategy they felt was possible; silence. This stance is frequently employed by families who cannot handle the truth. Another young woman who came to the work had been sexually assaulted by her older brother when she was very young, and her family's solution to them both having to live in the same house was to put a lock on her bedroom door and to lock the door that led from his room to hers. Nobody in their community knew a thing. Bea's abuse was known to all but never mentioned, and she alone had carried the weight throughout her life, critically affecting her intimate relationships with men. She was completely naïve to drugs of any kind and arrived tremulous to the place of consultation with a handwritten list of forty-three questions. When these had been addressed to her satisfaction, a session day was scheduled. In her first session, Bea lay quietly as the first dose approached her and then, having gone to the bathroom around ninety minutes, took the second dose. After ten minutes or so, she took off the eyeshades and sat up saying she felt sick. I went over to give her a bucket and sat beside her on the couch, my hand on her back. She retched, hating it, and then retched again. She then sat in utter stillness, staring vacantly for a moment or two, before suddenly declaring, "It's over! It's over!"

That was my story—but it is over now. My past is in the bucket! It can't touch me anymore.

I had many questions. The most important question was, "What if I were the perpetrator?" The answer was, "The truth will set you free." And it did.

A little over two years after that, I went for a second MDMA session to get some direction as to my purpose in life. Had I known the outcome, I never would have gone as I would not have thought that I was ready or even worthy.

Everybody is worthy; they just don't know it yet.

The miracle happened with only one dose, but I had to take the "blinders" (eyeshades) off to see. I experienced the "Glory of God," and saw that you have to totally surrender yourself to God in order to receive Him. And in my particular case, I saw that all my pain and suffering was a very small price to pay to see the "Glory of God on Earth." I am truly blessed as I believe most people spend their entire lives in fear and only see "the Light" before they die.

A deeply religious person throughout her life, Bea is forever grateful for her work with MDMA. She states the medicine does not lie. The medicine gives us nothing but ourselves, and in each of her two sessions, she received profound blessings.

First, she was disabused of the pernicious idea, carried by many victims of sexual abuse, that she herself, the victim, was the perpetrator. This odious notion is given to the victim by the perpetrator and is tragically aided and abetted by the appalling 'seduction theory' that is part of psychiatric orthodoxy, a craven formulation which proposes that it is the child who seduces the adult. This pernicious and utterly false notion has not only led to situations where the child's word is met with suspicion and denial, but it has contributed to acceptance of the 'false-memory syndrome,' a vile canard born of wilful ignorance and another facile denial of the truth. To have to carry not only the disgust from gross violations of oneself but also the shame from believing you were the perpetrator is a recipe for self-loathing.

Second, Bea experienced the gratuitous grace of Divine presence. No mortal could have contrived this, the most perfect corrective antidote for the feelings of doubt, fear, and self-disgust with which this righteous woman had unnecessarily lived her whole life. Many years post-session, these dreadful feelings have never returned. Deservedly, her past is truly in the bucket.

* * *

I was so afraid to bring a girl into the world.

C. F.

C. had done many years of talk therapy from when she was in college and as an adult, experiential work with breathwork. This experience of exploring within herself was preparatory to her single medicine session and served her well. Having some familiarity with the nature of her abuse, albeit incoherent and without details, the medicine allowed her to experience the deepest, darkest part of her psyche. The horror of what she had endured as a child became crystal clear, and it was this dreadful clarity that enabled her to be released from the emotional impact of her serial sexual abuse. Once the psyche understands that we are no longer caught and held within the horror and are comfortably and safely situated on a couch, it releases its hold.

When I was a child, I was in deep competition with my brother, who was three years older, and I tried to outdo him as much as I could, because I understood that he was getting more attention than I was, because he was the male. In high school, I was in every activity, in every play, was the regional president of my youth group that spanned five states, and on the newspaper. I was a straight A student. I was on the swim team; I was the head of the class; and I was on student council and on and on and on. I tried to get as many things behind my name as I could. I kind of had a mini-breakdown around junior year in high school, and I went to my guidance counsellor and said, "Look, I'm doing too much. I'm exhausted." His answer was, "Oh, just keep going. It'll be fine. You'll work it out," and I did. That was my mode for most of my life: Work, work, and just keep working and ignore all the feelings and just excel, and everything will be fine. That same guidance counsellor tried to hit on me in front of his wife when I ran into him again five years later at a friend's wedding.

When I was in college, I rebelled and got involved in the night life in a way I hadn't before. I was disenfranchised with my Jewish religion, didn't want to join a sorority and started hanging out with the Goth crowd and some bad boys. I ended up being very promiscuous. I was having sex a lot with guys I didn't like and was not protecting myself. I thought I owed it to them. I would get into these circumstances over and over again, where I would go way further than I wanted and felt like I had no control or no power in the situation. As I was coming out of college in my senior year, I said to myself, "You know what?" I heard what other people were talking about and their stories about their boyfriends and their lives, and I thought, "This is not what my experience is. I'm having a very different experience that doesn't feel good at all. Something must be really wrong." I went to a therapist of the university. The first therapist I went to was not helpful. He encouraged me to, "Keep going and find somebody that you like."

I started to research what was happening to me. What does it mean that I was promiscuous and not taking care of myself? I felt no control and was working so much and hiding all of my feelings. From the books I was reading, it became clear quickly that I was acting like a sexual abuse survivor. Still, I didn't really have any memories of anything happening. There were just fragments of weird memories that I hadn't categorised before.

I'm grateful to my mother who was in therapy at the time and had been in therapy for quite a while dealing with her parents and trying to understand the relationship in order to better figure out how to respond to them. She sent me to her therapist and encouraged me to figure out what was going on with me. I did some Gestalt therapy with my mom's therapist and with a group, and that was where my research further confirmed that I'd been sexually abused, or I was acting like somebody who had been. That kind of started my journey to understanding, healing, becoming whole, trying to understand what I really wanted to do, and what I liked, instead of just competing with my brother.

I moved away from my parents and hometown. In the new city, I studied Peruvian shamanism, was part of a women's therapy group and did traditional therapy work. I also explored as many alternative modalities as possible, including looking at past life regression, mediumship, healing circles, Tai Chi, yoga, massage, and more. It was all helpful. I started to retrace my childhood memories and place them in this new context. I realised at that point that the "kind of" sexual relationship with my brother that I had kept secret for so long and tried not to think about probably was connected in some way to my revelations about my current behaviour. I'd had sort of a sexual relationship with him. Later in life, when I got up the courage to ask him about it, he said, "Well, you were kind of the one that instigated that," even though I was three years younger. I was angry about that for many years, and then I became curious about it. "Wait, I'm three years younger. How could I have instigated that? What are you talking about?" What happened between us was kind of like side-by-side sexual play or curiosity. He wasn't really interested in doing anything *with* me—he turned out to be gay—but I really wanted him to be interested in doing it with me. This created feelings of not being good enough. I wasn't attractive enough. I didn't have all the things that were needed to be wanted. It was really important for me to be wanted, another sign of being sexually abused. Why would that be so important to me? Maybe that's what girls go through today, I don't know.

In my late twenties, I started to do breathwork and got more glimpses of the relationships in my family, with my uncles, cousins, grandfather, and with my father. It wasn't like there was anything overt that had happened, but it was kind of all a little over the line of too affectionate, too wanting to know what was going on in my personal life, too many uncomfortable looks, just a little bit inappropriate. I remember my grandfather on my mom's side said—I was sixteen and I had fishnet stockings and a dress on—"Look how sexy you look; you could be in *Playboy*." My mother was there, and she got angry with him and said to him, "That's inappropriate; never say that again. Hello? What were you thinking?" I knew I was defended, and that felt good.

I had all those pieces. I did a lot of work in breathwork around healing that and forgiving my mother. I told my mom about what I was realising, and she said, "I'm so sorry. I'm so sorry. I knew that it was over the edge, but I felt like I couldn't do anything, and I so apologise for that today." That was really helpful and confirming. My father's been pretty dismissive of the whole thing, but I would say that recently I'm realising that maybe he didn't do anything overtly but maybe covertly; there's something going on there.

Breathwork also led me to being able to heal so much with my father, forgiving him for whatever he grew up with, and whatever his role was in my abuse. My mom's father was abusive to her mother, and I think the same with my father's side, so I did a lot of letting go of that. Then, after years of breathwork, I heard about the MDMA work.

In the session, what came to light was something I'd had glimpses of in little bits. It was that my dentist and his wife or dental assistant had sexually abused me from the ages of seven to eleven, while I was coming to the dentist. There was a door between my mom out in the waiting room and me sitting in the dentist's room, so she could not see what was going on. I realised that I'd been threatened with my life, with a sharp dental instrument against my neck. If I told anybody, I would die.

Then, after several years, they started to say, "If you tell anybody, we'll kill your family." He would abuse me. The dentist would have sex or even actually sodomise me. Also, he would use instruments and put those inside of me, or he would have sex with his assistant and want me to watch that, and then sometimes, there was another little girl there but not very often. This was how I learned what it looks like to be sexy, and what it is to be wanted, and what you should do to make yourself attractive, etc.

This was not as clear in the memory, but there was some kind of back room. Some other guy was there. He was bigger and meaner. He was much more forceful, and there were little boys there, too, and I think he would sodomise all of us, but I don't think that happened very often. There would be a door locked, and we couldn't get out. That was kind of what was happening in the session with the MDMA, that feeling of not getting out the door and being stuck in there with him and being really scared.

There were other pieces that came out there, too, that made so much sense for me in my life now, which is that I think they tried to either start my period or stop it with medication. They also never actually cleaned my teeth. I have horrible gums and teeth to this day. Although, they would pretend that I had cavities or something and have me come in extra times. Also, my breasts didn't grow correctly. I don't have enough breast tissue. When I had my first baby, I had a lot of depression around that, because my breasts were not fully formed. I'm not sure what exactly happened with that, but it was part of the trauma.

Seeing the images in the MDMA experience was a huge relief. I could begin to understand and see what the situation was and what I'd been thinking. I'd had some fragments of memories of some kind of trauma in the dentist chair. Every time I got in the dentist's chair for the rest of my life, I'd have major anxiety. I also had glimpses of the blinding light they used. I only had these fragments of it, so the MDMA content kind of filled in the puzzle. I was relieved. It was a feeling like, "Oh, my gosh, okay. Now, I understand. Now, I have the pieces."

Even if this isn't exactly what happened, it makes so much sense that I'm holding the energy of this and the gestalt of it. I did holotropic breathwork a month or so later. And through the whole session, I wept and wept and wept for my little girl and for myself. I actually was able to visually tear down the walls of the story of the dentist's office, remember all of the trauma, and forgive everyone involved—the dentist, the assistant, and that guy behind the door. I also forgave my parents for whatever role they had too. I knocked those walls down and embraced my family; I walked away toward something better. It was hugely healing and hugely effective in being able to move forward.

It all helped me to make these big changes in my life. I've let go of a job where I'd been subtly abused by a woman who was my boss, who I love and is a great friend of mine, but was also dysfunctional. I left that after twenty years. I've done more holotropic breathwork since then and continue to realise more about the sodomy abuse. These were things that hadn't come out of my MDMA session.

As a child, I was extremely constipated, and I thought that my constipation was what caused my anal fissures. One particular breathwork session made me realise that I was constipated, because I was cut and hurt from being abused, not the other way around. I lived with that for so many years. I had such painful bowel movements and the bleeding and all that. I remember in the MDMA session that I'd had blood in my underwear at the dentist's office, and the dentist's assistant told me she loved me and to go hide it at the bottom of the garbage at home and not to tell anybody, because they'd threaten me. It was kind of that mixed-up love.

My whole childhood was sexualised, as well. There were weird sexual things going on with kids in the neighbourhood. One girl next door slept over, and I thought that she had been wanting to be kind of sexual with me. I was probably only nine or ten. Later, I realised that it might have been me starting it, because of what I'd learned, and what I thought it was to be a girl. My father also had *Playboy* magazines in his bedroom, and my brother and I looked at those. That was part of that situation with him. Then, there was another girl in the neighbourhood; we were getting naked behind the bushes and playing, and when the mother found us, she completely shamed me and told me that I could never play with her daughter again. She said, "How dare you!" That was the last time I played with her.

This was all happening during the years I was being abused at the dentist's office. This was happening between second and sixth grade. I used to have long beautiful hair, and I wore fun outfits, but during this period, I got a bowl cut and glasses and started to dress differently, because I was trying to hide.

This work has shown me how sad I was for myself when I was a little girl, and how sad I am for my daughter, who I had so much trouble bringing into the world, literally. When she was born, she had warrior badges on her forehead, scrapes and blood scars, because she was stuck. I was so afraid to bring a girl into the world.

I would say that the MDMA work brought everything to such clarity and such continuity. There were so many pieces of things that I didn't understand. The MDMA helped me piece it all together and have a much broader view of what had happened, and why I was the way I was, and how I could let that go and continue to heal. And, yet, at the same time, I really feel like I'm kind of a vessel. I'm an open person, and hopefully I'm healing for the ages and not just for me.

I feel like it answered so many questions that I have been able to let go of much of it. I know now that I'm not crazy. Again, I thought they were all kind of separate pieces, but seeing them all together makes so much sense, and I can just forgive myself more, which I've been doing a lot. I can be in the world differently, and I'm also seeing how I'm relating differently to men, I believe. I think I sexualised them, as well. That's what I learned, right?

In high school, I didn't have any boyfriends, but I did sexualise those boys. I had these horrific continuous crushes on so many of them; so many of them that didn't turn into anything. And then I swung the other way in college and was completely promiscuous while still having these crazy crushes on men. The crushes continued for a long time, despite being married and loving my husband. My whole view of sexuality and relationships has been skewed most of my life. I feel like I'm in a different place with that now, somewhat. Again, time will tell, but I want to have a healthy view of both men and women and be in a healthy relationship with it all. That's my goal. I think this work, the MDMA work, is helping tremendously to be able to do that.

Before MDMA, all these pieces were flying around, and I didn't understand how my behaviour related. Realising these terrible events has made my feeling about myself more coherent. Now, I can see, "This happened, so I behaved like this," rather than assuming, "I'm behaving like I'm crazy. What the hell happened?" Knowing the details, as awful as they are, has made it possible to see it as something that happened to me rather than something that's wrong with me.

I think the MDMA is wonderful, because it enables you to get into the very darkest pieces of it. I think that was incredibly helpful to be able to see the whole picture and that's probably why I didn't see it before, because it was just too painful. I didn't have the guard between me and it that the MDMA gave me. I think the

MDMA provides that in a wonderful way. I am grateful to have been able to see and integrate and take in the truth in what has turned out to be the most loving way.

Forgiveness is always a singular act of grace and courage but in this instance, considering the unbelievable vileness of the abuse perpetrated on this child over many years, forgiveness of the perpetrators is an extraordinarily open-hearted and generous act. It speaks of an understanding built into many specific biographical experiences in non-ordinary consciousness that include a sensation of the infinite, the experience of the small that also includes the large. Within this sensibility we are given to understand the frailty of all human beings, their weaknesses and their divine flaws, enabling forgiveness.

Forgetting is not an option, however, and recall of events made explicit through involvement with MDMA becomes, post-session, a normative process of retrieval from long-term memory. Only when the truth is known, when we can finally understand that we were grossly violated and played no part in the events except as victim, are we relieved of the odious idea that something is wrong with us. What is lost is the fear, the emotional charge from the events; it was simply disgusting, but now it's over, done and dusted, thank you very much.

● ● ●

I am home and tomorrow is a new day.

McKayla V.

Sometimes a client will come to the work from a great distance and in-person follow-up is compromised. It was by a rare chance encounter that McKayla was introduced to the possibility of healing with MDMA, but once she had heard about it, she went to great lengths to bring herself to the work. She had grown up in a family with six older brothers, and her designated role was scapegoat. As a young woman, she had married an abusive man who died of cancer, leaving her to look after their son with little financial support. The following is an e-mail exchange between her attendant (A.) and herself as client (C.) the day following her session, describing her difficulty engaging with her brother, the most agreeable family member and the one with whom she had chosen to stay. She experiences her brother's blaming and scapegoating of her, exactly as he and her family had done for years; but here, through the power of simple mindfulness, she sees in real-time right in front of her eyes what is happening, calls him out on it and, ta-da, the old-old story starts over again. Seeing the underlying pathological struc-

tures beneath our behaviour and their behaviour may be difficult, but it is a real head-start toward any ongoing inner work and very worthwhile. Only one party needs to change in order for any relationship to change.

C: Sorry to bother you again.

A: It's good to hear from you.

C: Wished I had stayed to talk with you a bit longer like I wanted to on that Friday, but I wanted to get to my son, a habit of mine, but regret ignoring what I was feeling in wanting to stay awhile longer.

A: Understood.

C: I have a question. I was told (by another attendant) I should find someone supportive to be with the following days after. Having this complex PTSD has stolen a lot from me, and I have isolated myself for many, many years and have no one I am all that close with.

A: Perhaps you might consider becoming involved in some activities at church; your faith has meant so much to you, and I could imagine you might find some folk there, if not 100 percent on your wavelength, at least agreeable. Being around such people can be a good way of resetting our habitual reactions from our belief that we are the scapegoat.

C: I only speak to this one brother and stayed with him, which turned out wasn't the best choice at all. He is a very anxious and nervous person. At first, I could notice and just observe, but then

I started to become very nervous, anxious, and angry. My anger got triggered, because I feel he noticed a big difference in me and was almost ruining it for me. He wasn't all that supportive but consumed with himself and a nervous wreck. It got to me, and I was triggered.

A: I'm sorry you got triggered from being in this situation, which was not ideal. However, apart from the difficulty at the time, no worries at all. Over time, you will be better able to avoid 1.) the situation and 2.) the need to respond (which I submit was simply habitual).

C: Does this mean by being around someone with my family drama has set me back?

A: No. It was only interrupted and not allowed to become integrated at that time. The fact that you are witness to this experience, this all-too-familiar insult to your identity and integrity, is what is important. Blaming yourself is how you have habitually responded to such events, but the beauty is that you now see yourself doing this at the moment it happens and can therefore make moves to change from blaming yourself to something closer to the truth.

C: I felt like my transcendence was being broken into, and I was thinking I would have been better off alone and pondering and relaxing by myself and with my son. I am leaving today and am hoping that this has not ruined anything for me?

A: Not at all, and by being such a cruel hit that you have owned, it may make you stronger. As I say, the work is a gift, and then the real work starts.

c: I can get back on my path to recovery that I did feel I was on?

a: And you are still on your path. As painful as it must have been for you with your brother, it alters nothing about the insights you had, nor does it diminish or affect your ability to integrate these going forward.

c: Has anyone else you know ever been flung into family drama soon after?

a: Yes, it is a must to avoid, and I regret that you got hammered.

c: I mean, at this moment, my intense anger and nervousness of never feeling loved or nurtured isn't lingering as long as it used to, which I guess is a good sign.

a: It absolutely is, and you can trust that this is now established within your psychic worldview.

c: But I still got triggered shortly thereafter?

a: In truth, this is merely a bump on a log; it sucks but is not going to de-rail anything you have experienced.

c: Is this what you meant that it's too much to ask ourselves what has happened, and that it still can be unfolding as some time passes?

a: This is part of that. We need to understand what has occurred, but to expect we can do this at the time of the session may be asking too much. But nothing is lost, and by keeping your experience in your heart and by bringing it to mind as often as you like, you will be doing everything possible to integrate it. Your stay with your brother was less than ideal, so let it be a teachable moment and find other places to stay; I can help. If you feel comfortable, call me.

C: Perhaps tomorrow? And it will not bother.

A: With respect, the very idea of 'bother' is your old self creeping back; you used it at the beginning, and it is a deeply embedded part of your operational stance in the world, the 'idea' that you are a bother. I am happy to help you make the best use of the courageous work you did here.

C: I will do my best to just relax into it until some time passes with the possibility of meeting again.

The exchange above resulted in a follow-up e-mail the next day:

Oh, gosh, I am so glad I went ahead and asked you about my concerns. It's like you were there or something. He did, in fact, scapegoat me when I approached him about his nervousness and uptightness, and how it was wearing on me a little. I had some things come up, and some discoveries weren't so good that I would have liked a listening, caring ear. I had only got around to telling the good stuff, but after that he was too nervous. When I mentioned his nervous uptight behaviour and was wondering what the heck was going on, he did, in fact, turn around and start to blame me for it. I was shocked, because I was in a pretty good mood and very calm, so why am I to blame for his nervousness?

But I truly held my ground and told him he was blaming me, and I wasn't going to accept that again, and he backed down after a while. I have come to the realisation that my family does not want what's best for me. He too has been trained to scapegoat me. I started to do well, and it made him nervous, because he was not used to seeing me like this or talking like this, and it made him so nervous, because he had to look at himself now and didn't want to look at himself; he just wanted to throw it on me. I finally didn't carry it. But it was really upsetting and confusing, because I thought he was the one family member who did care, although I still think he might have an agenda, and I don't trust him completely. The other reason was because he was the one who helped me research about things that can help PTSD, so why he wasn't all that happy for me was beyond my understanding.

I think your suggestion about the going down to the church activities is a great one. I was very hurt by my brother, and I also had the fear of being alone creep in, but I am now managing a bit better, especially now that I made it to my safe surroundings at home and landed safely. And especially after reading your very encouraging and helpful e-mail. I thought of church activities too but kept putting it off, but now I am going to, because I told my brother, "I need to heal, and I take my journey in trying to heal my complex PTSD very seriously." I think we need some time to NOT talk anymore for a while. He was the last family member I had hope for, and it really hurts that he is still in that sick family unit. Loss of the last family member hurts, but it hurts more to be scapegoated, and I told him it's so much more important for me to just work on my health now.

So, you are correct again about me saying those things about bothering you and apologising. I have done that to my family, my whole life, and to other people. I do have those fears, and I guess they are ingrained and are more false beliefs. But this time,

I noticed after the fact and don't normally even do that. So glad you pointed that out as well. Another bad habit is portraying myself in that way when I don't need to. I definitely did all the apologising and overly so at times. I apologised when someone hurt me in my family. But of course, I never got an apology ever from anyone, which is where the devaluing and belittling comes in. I am trying my best to break that, because I don't want my son to pick up on how much I sometimes apologise too much, even when I don't have to; I know now and am starting to become more aware of what my state transmits.

I am home, and tomorrow is a new day. Once again, completely grateful for your response; it was so much what I needed to hear. The insight is remarkable how you pick up everything to the tee.

And that quote you sent was excellent; thank you for sending. I totally understand it and get what it is saying, because I am living it. It is helpful to know you're not alone in that same feeling, and it was so well put down. So, thank you for that as well. It did help.

Well, it's off to sleep and thank you again. I really feel like I would love to send you a nice plant or something for your place. You have just been so great for getting me through this process, and I am so totally grateful.

The quote to which McKayla refers was from an ongoing correspondence this attendant was having with another client who has spent many fruitful hours on the couch and is fascinated by the workings of the medicine. He wrote, "My inner nerd is attempting to explain a theory of trauma and how the identity (ego) appears to diminish or retreat with an analogy somewhat similar to the function of a modern-day dimmer (for lighting). Rheostats worked on a differ-

ent principle that involved an adjustable degree of resistance, thus reducing flow of electrons. But newer dimmers turn current on and off so rapidly that the eye cannot detect. I think it's possible that the mind simply gets caught in a non-resolving cycle of, "I'm OK; I'm not OK," like the on-off of a dimmer. There is no actual split in our psyche, but the dimming effect is similar to loss of presence very much like dissociation. I guess the rapid on-off is similar to hyper-vigilance. The medicine work seems to allow one to slow down the on-off function to the degree that we can actually see the original alarm and correct the over-reaction. Kind of like resetting a gyro." This is an interesting hypothesis, but the full understanding of the psyche's mechanism-of-action of capture and release must await the possibility of future empirical research post-prohibition.

During her first session, I looked over to see McKayla tap her forehead repeatedly with her forefinger, reminiscent of the, "I coulda had a V-8" gesture. She writes, "I remember the most remarkable thing was when I sat up and whipped off my mask in amazement, and my eyes were probably like a deer caught in headlights. I saw you looking straight at me, and before I even said anything, you said with a very calm slight grin, "It's all a lie." I'll never forget that. It was as if you knew what I was experiencing, and I hadn't even told you yet about the unplugging." She then demonstrated what she had been up to on the inside. Holding her arms outstretched and making two fists directly in front of her, thumbs touching, she quickly pulled her fists apart and made a "Pop!" sound. Repeat. Repeat. Repeat. The gesture was one of forcibly disconnecting herself from each abusive member of her family—mother, father, brother, etc. As she puts it, "I remember not only unplugging sockets of abusive family members but unplugging false beliefs. I was yanking apart many, many wires all over the place." McKayla gets emotional when she recalls the work she did and says, "It's not all peaches and cream perfect for me, but

*it is much, much, much better." She is continuing the work with a
local attendant.*

• • •

I was disposable in every sense of the word.

Alice P.

Alice had applied to be included as a subject in a university hospital study but was not accepted because her profile did not fit their exclusion criteria. Her desperation led her outside her comfort zone, so she came to work with us, and her courage, tenacity, and determination have been rewarded. When someone presents at the consultation, it is impossible to know what the trajectory or content of their sessions might be, but she specifically referenced a rape/kidnap in her thirties. However, Alice's work unfolded with increasing evidence of relentless, wall-to-wall abuse that rose, in its completeness, to sadistic levels. From her infancy, she had suffered and endured life-threatening behaviour from the only people she knew—her parents.

I have had a somewhat traumatic life as a child and some traumatic events as an adult. I would say that I've tried to cope with them throughout my adult life with therapy, many, many years of therapy and antidepressant drugs. I have been plagued with a sense of overwhelming fear and anxiety my whole life, and I had very low self-esteem. I just felt like therapy really wasn't helping, and antidepressants really weren't doing the trick; I felt very hopeless and very despairing. I heard a little bit about MDMA therapy. For somebody who has never tried any drugs, or even experimented when I was a young person, it felt like a huge leap to try it.

Out of total desperation, I thought I would. I really had nothing to lose at that point. I certainly trusted the legitimacy of the work and the practitioners. I didn't feel like I was jumping off a cliff, but I think it was just desperation and despair, because I am very conscious of the fact that it's not considered a legal avenue. It was total desperation that pushed me to it.

After my consultation, I was still very fearful of it, but I guess I had enough trust in the research that I had read, and the fact that they were following protocols, I thought I'd give it a try.

I think I had six sessions altogether. The first one was very powerful, and it felt like an awakening and an opening. It really felt mostly like an opening and a beginning of understanding things, but the remaining sessions became very, very troublesome, and very dark. I had a very, very difficult time processing them and coming to terms with the memories and the images. It was a very hard year, but I think from each of those sessions, once I got through the trauma after maybe two or three weeks, it really felt like some things were beginning to heal, and that some clarity was starting to enter my consciousness. I had a much better vision and understanding of who I was. It was almost like my brain, or my memories, or my emotions, were like a tangled ball of yarn and that they're gradually loosening up and opening up into a pattern, like a knitted pattern, so to speak. Then, I could see some pattern of who I was there.

The first one turned out to be one of the milder ones, looking at it in perspective. That one was easier to handle than some of the others. There were a couple of facets to it. One is knowing what happened, and two is accepting that it could have happened. Then comes bringing it into the continuum from the past to the present and understanding the effects that those awful events had on me, and how they impacted me my whole life. I really didn't see it. I knew I was fearful, and I knew I was frightened. I knew I was angry, but I didn't understand the bigger picture. Now, I can see much more clearly how it affected basically my sense of self-worth for my entire life and how the lack of self-worth and self-esteem just constrained and limited my life.

I can also see a lot of things in myself that I did to hurt myself or where I hurt other people, that I don't think I could really see that clearly before, because I was just trying to deal with the fear. I couldn't really understand my reaction to that fear, the consequences of it.

I think the sad part is that I don't think I was ever a happy, pretty little girl. I think the abuse started when I was very, very young. I know it, because the things that my mother said to me about me being an unlovable baby, and an un-cuddly baby, and all of those things. Realising I was a baby who never cried and who never asked for anything, even as an infant, makes me realise that it must have really started from early infancy. I remember, even when I was a very young child, people saying, "Why is your little girl so unhappy? Why are you so sad?" I don't think I ever had any real happiness as a child. I do remember one time being with an aunt who bought me a toy. I was so overwhelmed, but I was so ashamed, because I didn't know what I was supposed to do with it. I didn't know what I was supposed to do in return for it, how I was supposed to pay her back. It became a very troubling event. I wasn't able to take in any happiness or joy. I was always just looking how to prevent abuse.

I was hypervigilant from very early on, I realise now. What I realised is how it's very hard for me to connect to people, because it's so hard for me to trust them. I'm always wondering what they're going to do to me, even now. Even intellectually, I know there are good, kind people in the world. It takes me a long time to really determine whether a person is a good, kind person. I have in my life chosen to be with a lot of very harmful, abusive people, not even realising they were, but just because that was my pattern.

I didn't really know how to see evil or more than that, I think maybe I just never learned to trust my instincts, because I think I was so abused. When I would question it or protest, my mother or my father would say, "That's not true, we love you. We're doing this, because we love you, et cetera, et cetera." I never really learned to trust my instincts that told me these things were wrong. Certainly, all the men in my life have been very abusive.

I think I always knew that I was disposable. During my sessions, I remembered my mother beating my head against the bathroom floor, and I had the thought that she could kill me. That memory was at three years old. The knowledge that my mother could kill me...I would always be conditioned by that knowledge. I was a burden. I had to earn my worth; I had to somehow earn it by doing all these awful things they wanted me to do.

There was a lot of sexual abuse. There's a lot of awful stuff, yes, so awful I can't even talk about it. There was just a lifetime of abuse. When I turned sixteen or seventeen, I think I was just going off the deep end, and I couldn't be abused any more. That's when my mother just sent me away. She just disowned me. I was disposable in every sense of the word.

She just basically said, "I don't want you. I'm going to send you back to your father." He didn't want me either, so it was like I didn't belong anyplace, and nobody really wanted me. I think I just felt like a very unloved, unlovable person. I think, even to this day, I live a very lonely, isolated life because of that.

I would say that the outcomes of doing the work have been productive. I would say that it's been a healing process. It's been a process of understanding myself, a process of reclaiming myself and really trying to learn who I am, and what I might want. I'm still struggling with this, and I still have a very, very long way to go. I think my big thing is that I have to come to the point where I believe I am a worthy human being. That is the essence of my struggle. I know what it is now. I don't know if I'll ever get to that point, but I think I know where I need to go now, whereas before I didn't know where I needed to go.

I don't think anybody loved me. For me, the challenge is to understand that it's not because I was unlovable. Even though I still feel like I'm unlovable, intellectually, I know that's not true.

People might look at me from the outside and say I've had a relatively successful life, which I would not agree with, but I think if I have accomplished anything professionally or educationally, et cetera, it's all been because I was trying to prove myself worthy and lovable. It was never as a self-fulfilling thing, or something I wanted to do, or something I enjoy doing. It was always just grasping at something to make myself worthy in other people's eyes.

I don't even like my job. I've studied things I didn't care about. It wasn't like I decided I wanted to do something. It was like, "Oh, my God, how can I make myself better?" I would just grab at anything that was available. It wasn't like I chose anything; I would just grab at whatever was there. I can't explain it.

What I did develop was extreme tenacity and determination, yes. I wouldn't say I have many other positive qualities, but those certainly were. I was very tenacious and determined. If I set my mind to something, I could do it, and I was smart. That was a blessing that helped me overcome a lot, because I was going to so many schools and things. I was changing schools. The only way I was able to succeed in school was because I was smart. That was a blessing.

I think the problem is that it's very hard for people to understand the truth about MDMA, because they haven't really experienced anything like it. I think that's the challenge. It's just such an unknown. It's hard to explain, and I think people are so afraid of these kinds of experiences in non-ordinary consciousness.

I look back and I think, "Oh, my God, what a wasted life, what a wasted life." I didn't really live. I battled with my fear; that was what my life was. Very interesting to look back at it that way. Anyway, I'm at the end of my life. I'm going to try to get to a place where I can at least enjoy something. That's my hope.

Not only was Alice's mortal life threatened as a child, her very soul was abused. Having no advocates within her family structure, she had no chance to create a coherent identity for herself, no way of knowing if the fear and anxiety she always felt was something in her or something she had been mendaciously gifted. The revelations of this truth resulted in many days or weeks of discomfort following each session, but she always landed on her feet and returned to continue the struggle to find a life for herself. Again, the complexity of unravelling developmental trauma is always challenging and release can seem to be incremental, but by staying with the process and returning to the work, she has found a significant level of release.

The rape/kidnap Alice referenced when we first met was dealt with in her first session, leading her to be able to access deeper memories of sexual abuse and sheer brutality during her childhood. This winding back led her to understand how utterly unprepared she was as a young adult to be able to make any value judgement about a man's intentions, leaving her vulnerable to the predation she suffered as a young woman. The toxic mixture of violence and premature sexualisation experienced as a developing child erased any capacity she had to feel alarm at the advances of her rapist/kidnapper until it was too late.

A friend and colleague of this attendant had worked as an intern in the Natural History Museum in New York, when she had been a student at Columbia University and sociologist Margaret Mead was the Museum's president. This was during the tumultuous late sixties when the Weather Underground, the Black Panthers, the SDS, and other groups were in high-profile opposition to the Vietnam War. My friend asked Dr. Mead what she thought was the element within America that could destroy the culture, to which she responded without hesitation, "The nuclear family." Witnessing the results of

behaviour within the families of individuals undergoing work with
MDMA, I would concur.

. . .

It was as if it was smoke.

A. M.

A. M. and her partner requested a session for themselves, so two of us, a man and woman, agreed to be their attendants. They had come together in midlife with blended-family issues in the forefront, but around ninety minutes after taking the first dose, A. M. suddenly sat bolt-upright on her daybed with a look on her face of absolute terror. As she described the scene she was experiencing, we assured her we would not leave her side and encouraged her simply to stay present for whatever had emerged. Within two minutes, maximum, the woman attendant asked, "Where is the fear now?" to which the client responded, "It's gone." To our witness, this was an example of the real-time release of trauma that this medicine allows, as swift and decisive as when the trauma was captured in the first instance.

A beloved, dear, trusted friend recommended MDMA, which set the stage. I had known this friend for twenty-two years, so he knew who I was. We had done group conversations and some journey-work before. We were no longer living near one another, and he suggested, "While you're in the city, why don't you meet this friend?" My partner and I decided we would. We had met when we were both in our fifties and come into the relationship with baggage that no longer supported us as individuals or as a couple, some of which we were aware and some we were not, but we were committed to living the day-to-day with as much open-heartedness as we could.

It was a whole new life. I had moved into the city, started a new job, and now had a commitment to this family situation; he had two kids and a crazy ex-wife. Throughout my life, I had focused on caring for children in the world but did not want my own children in the world. God had different plans for me, obviously. After a lifetime of doing development work supporting women and children, now I had to do it myself. Instant motherhood. It was hard. What was especially hard was dealing with what was always coming up—the emotions and the difficulty when one is feeling self-doubt and shame. All of that somehow bubbles up in a relationship with a person that you love, and you find yourself treating them terribly. It's almost like you give each other licence to torture the other when you get into a relationship.

We had committed ourselves to try not to do that. This introduction to MDMA was exactly that; trying. What I loved so much about the process was the beginning, the setting of the stage. Our attendants were very mindful and loving with the introductions, so it was just like old friends coming together. We began this journey with MDMA which, in the chronology of my personal and therefore relational healing, was an invaluable cornerstone for me.

My partner came into the session having had a very difficult experience with his ex-wife the night before. He was somewhat distracted, but we decided to do it anyway. His experience perhaps was a bit less intense, but mine was extraordinary. It allowed me to understand that fear was running my show. I just never fully understood that. I began to understand why my journeys start off very intense, and then they are full-on. They always were in Panavision colour as well as demanding emotionally, physically, and psychologically. It was a kaleidoscope of experience.

I never have a slow glide in. I go right into the experience, and the experience on this occasion was initially this: I was in World War II, and there were dozens of tanks coming at me. I didn't know if I was in Nazi Germany, but that's what it felt like. That was curious to me, because I don't think I have any connection to that. I sat up. I remembered those gun barrels just looking down at me. It just seemed like there were hundreds of them, and it was impossible for me to overcome any of them. They were tanks, World War II tanks. It didn't matter what I was seeing, as the enormous amount of fear made it feel impossible to understand. I couldn't manage it. It felt like it was all-enveloping. I felt, "I can't get through this. I have to surrender." There's the tricky point with me. When I feel overwhelmed by fear, I go first to victim; I surrender. And then I want to go to war. Everything inside of me, every protector, every guard, every sentinel wants to go to war to attack so that you die before I do.

My old strategy was to kill, strike first. But now there were too many; I couldn't adopt an old strategy. I could not be the same person. I could not adopt the same response. The situation would not allow it. I had to find another way.

One can't live in the world where you're always fighting back and one certainly can't live in a relationship like that. It was the first drawing back of the curtain where I could actually have awareness about what I was doing and not be terrified. Because of the medicine, the moment I felt terrified, I could observe what was happening. Instead of being a victim to the circumstances, I was an observer. I was a witness. Therefore, it wasn't going to get me, and the medicine was inviting me to learn and to heal.

There was also this unbelievably important moment when my attendants came over. I don't know if my face looked as frightened as I was feeling internally, but I received the kindness and the tenderness that I don't think I knew much of growing up. I was the last of four kids, and my father travelled a lot; it was always expected that I would just suck it up. That moment of tenderness and kindness in the session introduced this awareness that I didn't have to go to war. My attendant asked, "What's going on?" and I said, "I'm afraid. I have to stop." I really thought, "I have to stop, because I have to kill whoever is coming at me, or I have to stop the experience, because I don't want to go through it." My attendant said, "We will stay with you. Just stay with it and see what happens."

Instead of fight-or-flight, which has been hardwired into my DNA, I stayed. I could stay with the tenderness of the experience, and when I stayed with the fear, it was nothing. It just vanished. It was like, "Poof." It was as if it was smoke, like in the *Wizard of Oz*, when the witch just disappears, and the smoke vanishes.

For my whole life up until this time, this nothingness had me by the throat. The moment I felt the fear, my heart would close. I'd go to war; I'd burn bridges; I'd break up relationships. It didn't matter. I just needed to take care of and save myself. Then, I knew it was nothing. Nobody else did anything. It was me staying, so simply, staying and surrendering to the gift of what was being brought to me by my own intention, by my own will or psyche or heart. It was a clearing away of the oppression and fear and then a further understanding that this was really a gift it was surrendering

For the rest of the journey, the fear didn't go away, just like fear doesn't go away in everyday life. But it was a different experience with it. It was, "Oh, you again. Seriously?" Instead of spending time avoiding the experience or avoiding the fear, I experienced this place of grace. In this place of, "It's nothing," there was this eco-system of, "I can do it, because I have it within me." If not, I knew there were people in my life and in the world who would offer a handhold as I went through the experience.

My partner and I just spent the rest of the experience cuddling and connecting and fell into the day-to-day that we wanted. The exterior hadn't changed.

I know I live in a big city, and it's relentless. I have a demanding job, and I travel a lot. I have two kids to care for and all of that. That's going to be the constant. It was the interior that had changed. In that shifting, like a glacier, I now had this new material, this information that allows me to remember when I get into the same spot over and over again. I have a knowing, a practice, to meet and move through it.

I have a sense the fear has a boundary. It's just a story that I've generated. It's a story that I've made up about something that's going to happen to me until I can stop and investigate. I certainly have other tools that I use—a meditation practice, a prayer practice that I've used throughout my life. What this experience did was to give me a piece of information that I didn't have before.

It's a system of support one must give to oneself. Fear comes up now and I remember it's nothing. If it was a physical fear, such as a fire, I would know what to do, but the experience of emotional fear provided a handhold, a piece of information that I just didn't have before. That information allows me to explore when the fear comes up, using whatever tools that are available in that moment.

Curiously enough, sometimes the fear visits with less frequency, but sometimes it's bigger and more intense. Because the ante's up, it's almost as if my soul or my psyche is saying, 'Okay, you can take it.' And, I understand, "Okay, I got this."

It doesn't mean my partner and I don't argue, but when we fight, that's my signal that I'm afraid. Instead of going for the jugular and saying, "It's either you or me, and I'm not going down." I can say, "Okay, what is going on? What's really going on and is there anything really there? Or is it just my old story that I've slipped into again?" It's a circuit breaker for that habitual response that no longer supports me. When I was aged three, four, or five, maybe it did. Now, as a woman, I need other tools if I want to live a robust, vibrant life. I just need different tools.

Interestingly enough, the experience had guideposts but not guidelines. This experience was a gift that has repeatedly supported my ongoing journey.

The medicine allowed me to stay with myself, which is something I generally hadn't been able to do before. With the staying, the fear went away. It was nothing. It was air. I can remember thinking, "It's air." Afterward, I could meet this same fear in a new way. It was the gift I was giving myself, an opportunity for me to explore fear with a different response, and I sometimes am even able to respond to my fear with the same love and kindness that was shown to me.

I think we are given all the tools we need to go through life open-heartedly, vibrantly, and robustly. Then life happens, and we forget. We get scared. And, the journey is remembering; remembering what's underneath.

"It was as if it was smoke," and, "I can remember thinking, it's air."

These statements were made after A.M. encountered a powerful, hidden fear that she has carried all her life, symbolically represented as being surrounded by WWII tanks. We can hear in other testimonies, Sgt. K's for example, where the moment of release is described, but in this and Bea's testimony, it is as plain as a pikestaff to both client and attendants. The trauma has been caught and held since its capture; the trauma is presented (symbolically) in-session; the trauma is experienced and owned; the trauma is released.

This demonstrates the action of 'unexperienced experience' in real-time, and it is entirely generated by the body's own inner wisdom. We do not, ourselves, release; we are released. Our only, but critical, task is to show up for ourselves and submit to the healing potential of the medicine.

A. M. says that sometimes in life the fear is more intense, an artefact of our being open to feel it rather than to deny it and act it out in life, where her only strategy had been to go Darwinian and exhibit a classic fear-response—kill or be killed. When we have experienced this 'fear' in a medicine session and can recall experiencing that "it's air," we can discern the phantom nature of the fear consciously in our lives and take steps to manage it. We need to simply understand that the fear is not actually us, it is not who we are, and we have been made fearful at some point or points in our lives by events outside of us. We can then objectify it, which is key. It is also huge to be able to say, "Oh, You again." and experience the beast, even in its bigger, more intense manifestation post-session.

A. M. is able to engage mindfully with the traces of fear that re-emerge going forward, because the thing has lost its power and can be recalled as it is now, a normal memory. It has become "a gift that has repeatedly supported the ongoing journey."

CHAPTER THREE

The Consultation

———

"As is your desire, so is your will.

As is your will, so is your deed.

As is your deed, so is your destiny."

THE UPANISHADS

The attendants to this medicine work operate outside the mainstream, but people who have exhausted every other option to ameliorate their condition do find their way to us, and many come with various levels of information (and misinformation) gleaned from word of mouth and their own research. Most clients approach the consultation, which must precede any consideration of actual medicine work, through references from friends who have done the work themselves and shared their experience. They have already done their due diligence, consulted internet sources, books and articles, as well as empirical studies like Dr. Mithoefer's.

It is important to note clients make their way to the work in order to heal, never as a form of recreation. It is a means to this end, not an end in itself. People come to us, because they have a problem or condition that has beset them for years, even decades, correctly described as "treatment-resistant." They cannot shake it with regular therapy, conventional psychopharmacological agents, or any other work they might be doing.

This first meeting is held in the same location where the work will occur with the same attendant who will be conducting the session. The first and most important step is to familiarise the client with how the session day will proceed and what may or may not happen during the experience. Trust is of foundational importance to this work, and no session can be considered if any doubts of this nature remain between the participants. The introductory consultation determines whether the client and attendant feel there is sufficient trust between each other, the work, and everything else to be able to commit to a session day.

Arriving at the consultation is, by itself, an act of quiet courage.

By definition, traumatised people are victims; they have gone through life as a victim, but by approaching the healing potential of MDMA, they demonstrate a readiness to change. The movement from a victim mindset to a more empowered "warrior" mindset is a critical part of beginning this work.

SET AND SETTING

Included in the consultation are considerations of the two essential factors to all work in non-ordinary consciousness since such work began in the 1950s; Set and Setting.

SET

The client's mindset, their "set" as they approach the work, is crucial. We need to know they want to do this work; it is not enough that their friend, brother, or spouse recommends it. The client, her- or himself, must be committed. Part of the initial consultation is devoted to evaluating and establishing their motivation and to ensure they are truly ready to do the work. If they are thinking along the lines of, "I have had enough. I need to move toward releasing whatever it is that is contorted within me and making me dysfunctional. If I can release the wounds with this work, I will do so," then they are thinking outside the victim box and moving toward becoming a warrior. They are committed to remaining open to whatever emerges, determined, in Mary Oliver's poetic phrase, "to save the only life that you could save."

SETTING

In the consultation, the attendant and client take time getting to know each other, deciding together that this is something they want to go forward with. Clients use the consultation time to become familiar with the space where they will be working, whether in the client's home or a pre-assigned location that is new to both client and attendant. The room layout ideally includes a long, comfortable couch with blankets and pillows, where they can stretch out for the afternoon. One client, a writer and admitted sedentary, stretched out in mid-session into a pose like Marilyn Monroe's first centrefold in *Playboy* magazine and exclaimed, "Who knew there was so much body!" The attendant sits in a chair adjacent to, but not right on top of, the client. We do not face each other but they know we are absolutely present for them. We are always within arms' reach, so if the client needs a hand to hold, we are there. It is a modified version of the classic setup used in psychoanalysis, with the patient on a couch and the therapist sitting behind them.

The client is encouraged to wear eyeshades (which can be removed at any time) for the duration of the session, so they can be out of eye contact for hours. Donning eyeshades also clearly signals the direction of the client's focus: Inward. One client later joked about his trepidation upon lying down with the eyeshades on, waiting for the medicine to take hold. He was thinking, "I hope he's not going to harvest my organs." The only reason he could joke about it that way was because he knew he was safe.

THE SESSION

Along with preparing the immediate environment, the setting, we explain the trajectory of the session step by step. We make it plain to the client they own the room, they have absolute control, and nothing will happen externally without their express consent.

We meet around eleven o'clock in the morning and take time getting settled and comfortable. It is usually around noon when the client takes their first dose of MDMA, usually 125 mg, dons the eyeshades and lies back, all in one movement. From this moment on, silence reigns supreme.

In an industrial society, silence is not absolute, and we are beset with beeps, pings, and alarms from many commercial appliances, not to mention planes, trains, and automobiles and their attendant noise. The silence we seek is a low, ambient level of sweet, bright and delightful music through such composers as Handel, Albeniz, Dowland, Marin Marais, Hildegard von Bingen and others, like the incomparable el Hadra, that serve to mask any intrusive sounds beyond our control.

For the first forty-five minutes to an hour, we do not move, speak, or make noise, giving the initial dose ample opportunity to affect the client. Between sixty and ninety minutes after administration of the first dose, the second dose, 75 mg, becomes available. There's no obligation to take it. Though some people find 125 mg to be adequate and useful, most do take the second dose, extending the session from four hours to five or six hours.

We explain, by taking the medicine, the client's work is done; they have nothing to do in the session. People sometimes assume there's a "right" way to conduct themselves, but the most productive strategy is to relax, be as open and receptive as possible, allowing the medicine to approach them. That surrender is crucial and is only possible when there is absolute trust between client and attendant. We also suggest a potential attitude shift. For example, many of us who may have lived fearfully may justifiably feel frustrated and angry with whatever symptoms bother us;

insomnia, anxiety, depression and so on. We may hate everything to do with our condition and project this feeling onto everything that comes up, hating the fear or anxiety itself. However, it behooves us to understand that the foregoing depredations are symptoms, artefacts thrown up by the body as messages to tell us something. "Hey, over here! Pain. Headache. Anxiety." This biological action by the body is not against us, anything but. It is trying to help by informing us of the underlying condition producing the symptoms of pain, headache, or anxiety.

We explain to the potential client in the consultation that whatever is bothering them does not want to be bothering them. The psyche took control and captured the traumatic memory in the first instance on our behalf, to protect us; it acted per its biological imperative to keep us whole.

With this in mind, we ask clients to consider a more nuanced approach in regard to the anger they may feel toward their symptoms and, with an understanding of their genesis, ask them to do what they can to regard them with compassion. In other words, we ask them to love their 'enemies', the symptoms, and to understand that they exist only as a result of the action of the psyche in its original protective capture. The psyche acted for us, not against us. The symptoms we hate are the by-products of the psyche's original act, being expressed by the body in its ongoing attempt to: 1) inform us of the underlying conditions, and 2) to release them to whatever extent that it can. To our view, MDMA gives the body its finest opportunity to release the symptoms arising from trauma and PTSD.

This softening of our attitude can be likened to 'diplomacy, not war,' and comports more closely with the feeling-tone of the medicine; kind, patient, and loving.

Some clients come to this work with preconceived notions of what it is like to take a consciousness-expanding drug, usually coloured by recreational experiments in college, at a rave, or with a group of friends. They may never have experienced the medicine given with the care, attention, and singular support they will receive with us. Keeping complete focus on themselves during a session, having a "meeting with yourself," as Deepak Chopra says, is customarily a revelation.

THE BODY KNOWS

One woman, around forty, took both doses, up to 200 mg, but after two hours was on the couch getting nowhere. She then assumed the classic cross-legged meditation posture and within a few minutes felt the medicine's effects. She told us afterwards that she had been a DJ in the 1980s and '90s where the coin of the realm in the dance clubs was 'ecstasy'. She, however, was not dancing with abandon but in control of the music, a complicated task requiring split-second timing, full attention, and extreme dexterity. Her body had evoked this responsibility out of habituation when it surrendered to the MDMA in the session, maintaining her at a high level of competence, vigilance, and function per its imperative during her DJ years. This priming from the past disallowed the psyche from having access to anything but this duty. Subsequent to her DJ years, however, she had developed a serious meditation practice, so by assuming the meditative posture, her body then understood that her circumstance had changed, adjusted its control to match this change and allowed her to experience the medicine deeply.

It is all but impossible to describe the inner experience of MDMA to a client, particularly how the non-ordinary condition shifts our attention to reveal that which we cannot see. As Lucy V. observes in her testimony, an analogy may be found in stereograms, those wallpaper-like patterns that we are asked to stare at until a Bengal tiger appears. As we stare and stare, it seems impossible; there is no tiger there, but then, in one moment, there's the tiger. Not only can we see it as plain as a pikestaff, we cannot un-see it. In this medicine work, the action of the psyche to reveal its captured secrets is similarly swift and enduring.

In ordinary consciousness, we are productive; we think, function, walk and talk, making full use of our five senses to comprehend the world we inhabit. Sight, smell, taste, touch, and hearing are all outwardly directed, interpreting sounds and smells to determine their nature, discerning on our behalf between burned toast and a fire in the basement. In this medicine work, all our senses are fully operational, but we choose to focus our attention inward, engaging with our sixth sense, a catchall term for an awareness that includes intuition and extrasensory perception. This becomes our primary focus for the duration of the session, within which time the psyche has the opportunity to reveal something that we have been conditioned to overlook. Like the Bengal tiger, it simply appears.

In the non-ordinary state precipitated by this medicine, we have nothing to do but receive and feel the relaxation, openness, and love as it unfolds. The words 'non-ordinary consciousness' may sound a bit alarming to some people, even something to avoid, but in fact, we surrender to the possibility of non-ordinary consciousness every night when we sleep. Through our ability to dream, we know we have the evolutionary potential, arguably even the predisposition, to enter a different form of consciousness.

SITTING STILL

Our modus operandi is to give the medicine the maximum opportunity to inhabit the client. Our point of view derives from our experience, and our action and non-action expresses the best we can do is the least we can do. Put another way, the less we do, the more the client can do. We are the fire department, not the police department. We take a radical backseat, but one that is, at the same time, utterly and completely present for the client. It is like looking after a sick child; you sit with them, not necessarily interacting. You are there, and they draw comfort from knowing you are there. That knowing is a very big part of the support our clients receive. They understand they will be attended to during every minute of the session.

For many clients, their MDMA session represents the first time they have done any kind of work that has offered them full attention and support from somebody who has no agenda but who is totally on their side. It is a unique experience to have someone sit by without any attempt to influence the unfolding of events, simply being present to whatever arises. Such quietude runs counter to orthodox therapist's training to interact verbally with the client, and not surprisingly, it is unusual to behave this way in our society. Usually, when we are with someone in trouble, we think, "I should do something. I should say something. I should help this person." Not in this case.

There's a quote by Buddhist meditation teacher, Reginald A. Ray, who writes about *bodhisattvas*, enlightened beings, and their ability to enter a situation without a plan of engagement:

> *"The [attendant], rather than acting toward sentient beings based on his opinions of what is 'good' for them, knows that he does not know and can never know what sentient beings need. All he can do is watch and wait until he sees, with direct and*

unmediated insight, what is called for. Knowing that he does not know, he does not act prematurely. He waits until this moment discloses its secret, which is its definable appearance, it's 'call,' such as that may be."

The *bodhisattva* sits, watches, and listens, waiting to see what may be necessary or not necessary. We seek to achieve an equivalent posture of attentive presence and utter non-intervention in our work; doing not doing.

As attendants, we have no agenda except to support whatever emerges from the client. We do not follow the Jungian path, the Freudian path, or any other of the many paths in the field of psychiatry and psychotherapy. Similarly, we espouse no spiritual, religious, or philosophical doctrine. We sit in silence to the greatest extent possible, silence being, in fact, an apt description of the feeling-tone of the medicine itself. What we offer in the client's immediate external environment is the pure neutrality of the same silence they are experiencing internally under the influence of the medicine. It's an open space completely free of interference. We respect that place when we completely trust and respect the medicine, allowing it the greatest opportunity to open us and manifest its healing potential.

There is no way to know what a client will feel, or how the medicine will affect them, and the inner silence may lead to tumult. One client did a few sessions that repeatedly brought him to a place where he revisited the trauma of his father beating him when he was a young boy. On the couch, he re-experienced his father's brutality, and it showed in his bodily movements—his knees were up to his chest and his arms were held up to shield himself from the remembered blows.

Over time and with further work with MDMA, this client's sessions have become calmer and calmer as his body re-experiences and releases the trauma he had endured as a youngster, completing the traumatic cycle. He has gained significant insight into specific events in his childhood and the dysfunctional dynamics of his family system as an outcome of his medicine work. His body is no longer holding tight to the original insult.

The body's struggles are not always easy to witness, but as attendants, we have done our own work and know how the story unfolds; the only way out is through. We can observe the trauma dispassionately, because we know such movements are the body's way of releasing the horror of abuse. For the time-limited duration of the session, we are traversing a very tight passage, and observing a client's physical responses underscores how trauma is held within the body. What we see the body saying is, "I've been wanting to let go of this for years." The whole system has, up until now, been holding onto the "frozen present;" it is as though the trauma were suspended in aspic. Now, when the medicine finally allows the psyche to understand that the client is safe, the psyche softens and releases the trauma it had captured and has faithfully held onto for so long.

The quietude offered to the client gives them the best opportunity to have the meeting with themselves that allows and gives maximum opportunity to their introspection. They are being presented with elements from their biography without interference from any outside actor. As they finally have this intra-psychic meeting, often the first authentic meeting with their true selves, the medicine allows the traumatic material to emerge.

Even clients who arrive with some apprehension see the common sense of the process, once it is credibly explained to them. After they experience the medicine, they literally cannot imagine they could have achieved the insights in any other way, a sentiment expressed in many testimonies. This allows the client and the medicine to interact with each other over a period of hours, giving the psyche the finest opportunity to understand they are no longer under threat and to release the traumatic material from which they have been safeguarded.

Attendants have been through similar experiences in their own work, adding another layer to the client's trust. Every single person who is doing this work, either as attendant or client, has some element of trauma in their own biography. Each one of us has found considerable release from the dysfunctions that were so radically affecting our lives. We come from the same place as our clients: "It is time. I've got to do something about this."

Among our group, we try to match clients with attendants with whom they have something in common; we refer to one another. One couple, for example, healed their marriage through MDMA work and have become attendants; they work with clients who also want to do the work as a couple. If a woman presents with an intimation of sexual abuse in her past, she may prefer to work with a woman. Sometimes clients work with one or more different therapists at different times. We share very openly with prospective clients what we can offer, so we can ensure them the most fruitful medicine experience possible.

Apart from our sincere commitment to the non-interventionist approach, we have no agenda beyond wanting the client to be able to make the most of the opportunity from their exposure to MDMA, to encourage a productive session. We have found this hands-off approach results in the most beneficial outcomes.

I just can't put words to it, how nice it was having her there.

J. C.

The following testimonies were transcribed from two interviews with a newly married couple soon after the medicine sessions they embarked upon together. Their focus was not on the possibility that they would encounter trauma from within their biographies, but from a desire for personal growth and to find out how they could improve their understanding of life, and to address issues about how they could best blend their two families after divorce. Their composure in-session was entirely harmonious, reflecting their inner experiences, and our conversation immediately post-session found them full of ideas about how they would do this or that differently going forward as a result of the insights they had gained. The two testimonies follow each other.

I came to the work from three different places.

The first was, having got divorced, I decided to go through the Hoffman Process. It really started a journey for me in terms of learning more about myself, and who was I as a person, and how could I be the best possible person, which led me to some Jungian therapy work and led me to books like *The Untethered Soul*. Then, I met this woman, S., who'd been on a very similar journey post-divorce. She'd also gone to Hoffman, and we began to realise that we were on very similar paths and similar journeys. We went on this MDMA journey together. So, the first part of it was having wanted to go on this expedition together.

The second was a good friend of ours who had been through an experience and strongly encouraged us as part of our own work to go try it.

The third piece is I belong to this forum group that I've been a part of for the past fifteen years. It's really been a critical part of my life as we push each other to get deeper into our respective journeys. All these things, all three areas, kind of led up to what was our first journeying experience.

The first session, for both of us, was tentative. I think it was partly because we were both nervous not knowing, never having done anything like this before. It was driving down that morning, and S. really began to feel uncomfortable and she felt that I was kind of forcing her into something. Several hours before our sessions, we had a serious heart-to-heart around, are we really sure we want to be doing this? And what if there's permanent damage? Of course, we know there's not. I would say our frame of mind going into it was probably less than ideal. I think we went into it open, not expecting anything, but with a little bit of trepidation as well.

As we got into the session and the experience, the trepidation was completely overridden by the experience itself. We were both alert and kind of conscious of feeling; I'm not sure it was a paranoia, but a cautiousness. But as soon as we got into the experience, as we did the second dose, we were both just overwhelmed by the experience. I think it was really the second half of it that was so powerful for us. It was also a noticeable difference from our second session, but I think that the second half of our first session really proved to be just a fantastic, fantastic experience for both of us.

S., in fact, walked away from that first experience even more of a proponent than I was. That astounded me. She was the one who, a few weeks later, said, "I absolutely, positively want to do this again, but I want to do it now with much greater preparation, much greater intention, and have more in-depth conversations in advance of the session to prepare for it." She was really the one who drove that, and that's what made our second session just such a home run.

In revisiting the first session, I feel the experience changed me profoundly. Theologically, I felt different after that first session and that it had opened up pathways in my brain. Almost like I could feel things, new pathways forming in places where I had been blocked before, let go. All of a sudden, for a week or two or three after that, I just felt like this glow that stayed with me. A lot of anxiety and stresses I felt on certain topics in my life disappeared. I felt, for the first time, I could really walk forward in my life without having the voices as baggage. It was a spectacular experience.

I think S. felt something similar but probably not as profound as mine was. Her second session was much more profound than her first one. The big difference for both of us was that in the first session, we went into it with some trepidation, with our foot on the brake, like okay, let's be very careful. Let's not get out of control. We didn't really know. We were allowing the experience to drive us or to pull us along.

The second session was so different because of our pre-conversation and that we went in there with much more specific intention on the one or two topics that we really wanted to focus on. I think we both felt like in the second session we could essentially guide the ship a little bit more. It allowed for much greater confidence, a more directive experience. That made it just so powerful, so liberating for both of us. The second session was so much better than the first, but the first session for me was spectacular. I think S. really felt the second session for her was the complete home run.

For both session one and session two, we feel like we advanced the ball in our lives and in our minds so much that now we feel like we're moving onto the next level, the next round of topics for us. I must say that having S., there beside me on the opposite bed for session one and session two made it so…I just can't put words to it, how nice it was having her there.

It allowed for a level of trust and a kind of co-experience together with her. We have some friends who have tried the experience, but they didn't have their spouse with them, and we've both described how different it would be if our spouse did not participate with us. It's an experience that is almost impossible to describe to someone who's not done it. To have S. there just made the experience so much more rewarding and enjoyable for me.

It allows us both to be open to topics that used to be emotionally loaded for us, but it has also allowed both of us to let go of some of the power and energy of some of the inner voices that we've had in the past. It allowed our best selves to come out and to be able to enjoy our kids at a level that we haven't been able to do in the past. For both of us, we have had active, successful lives and to be able to let that go and now focus all our energy and effort on our kids has just been such a gift. We could not have done this a year ago.

We have not described for anyone that we went through this experience, and we probably won't do that with our kids, but they have noticed how happy and quiet we both seemed. I understand the impulse to share this, because it is so precious. But in some ways, I can see how with our kids, who have not been on this journey yet, might be put off by finding out that their parents did this experience. So, when the time is right, we're going to tell them.

In the meantime, for Christmas, we gave all six of our kids the option to go to either Mountain Trek or the Hoffman Process, whenever they want. We want to encourage them to experience their own life journey. Now that we have the insight of having done this, we want our kids to have the most fulfilling experience they can have in their life. We want to encourage them to go on their own life journeys now.

• • •

Sharing this was a huge piece of it.

S.C.

I've been kind of on a learning journey for the last five years or so, with a fair amount of intentionality around personal growth, so I have opened up my lens on that front. A good friend of ours told us about her experience with MDMA therapy and recommended it. To be perfectly honest, I was not all in, until probably the moment we sat down in the living room. I just kept saying, "You know, I'll have the conversation, then I'll decide whether I'm doing this." I really did not know what to expect. I'm just so glad I did it. It's just been an incredibly remarkable experience.

In the first session, I really didn't have any effect until the second dose. Initially, I don't know how long it was…it seemed like quite a while. I just sort of thought, "Well, that's okay. I'll just lay here and have a rest for the afternoon."

It just took me by surprise, the experience. The first time, I really didn't know what to expect. I didn't come in with a plan or thoughts or anything. I just sort of reclined on the couch and waited to see what would happen. I was definitely nervous. I had a fantastic experience, but I think the second time was much different for me. It felt like a quantum leap forward, in terms of having integrated into my system.

I think a big difference there was that fantastic conversation we had at the beginning of our session the second time, where we had a chance to really get some guidance about how to approach it, and we talked about what intentions we might be going into the session with. I think that just made it a completely different experience, along with the fact that I wasn't having the first-time jitters.

The second session, again, it was just so much about the conversation we had at the front-end, and just going into that experience with those thoughts about, "Okay, I've identified what it really is that I'm looking to have an opening on," and that our attendant walked us through following the waves of the experience. Just sort of talking through the process really changed things for me.

I feel, now, like I just had a huge...I don't know what to call it, a breakthrough, an opening. That's the first time I knew that I'd had a wonderful experience, that I felt myself sort of try and grab onto as the time passed. The second time, it felt more like it just settled right into my system.

What made it even better for me is that I have someone who I go talk to maybe once a month, so there was a kind of touchstone along the way, but the enormous insight for me was I went in there saying I feel like I have this low-level anxiety a lot of the time, but it's not really serving me. There's no big reason for it.

Right away, almost as soon as I started in on the experience, right away was this very clear picture of this tying into my ancestors. I have this family history tied to the Holocaust and to pogroms, and there's been a lot of anxiety embedded into my history. I had this very, very powerful experience of saying, "Thank you very much. You know, I no longer need your services." That is exactly the experience I had, of saying, "Wow! My ancestors have carried a lot to bring me to the place where I am today." I'm incredibly grateful to them, and the way to thank them for that is to not carry forward the anxiety. I don't need it anymore.

That really entered my system in a profound way. It was a feeling of general anxiety, like a physical sensation but also just a general 'on-guard.' Not to overstate it. I don't think I had anything that you would go to a doctor and get diagnosed. It was just something that was holding me back, and I feel like it's gone now.

The amazing thing, also, to me, is your psyche knows where it came from. I didn't go in there with that intellectual thought in my head. It just came, and it came immediately and was just so true. I've really come to embrace that concept very deeply, because I had several instances in the last handful of years where I never gave any thought to my ancestry at all, yet it's just come down to the fact that's where things come from. I think you can carry a lot of stuff with you.

I know a lot of people who come to this work are coming because they have some very present trauma in their lives. I think it's just interesting that I had such a powerful experience without that. I had a very sound, safe, loving upbringing. I am incredibly fortunate in my life. I've clearly got the same shit everybody else does, but I wasn't coming in there to get rid of some trauma I knew of, and yet look at all that was uncovered. I had this amazing opportunity to transform, even though I didn't have a big problem. It's just interesting to me that I could get that much out of it.

What makes this so important for me is all my work for the last five years does not feel like this is just about me feeling better. It is about me feeling like I am doing my best, most powerful work. I work in the space of social justice and kind of play my part in making the world better. On behalf of my family and my relationships, it felt like it was an incredible gift to me, but that the most important thing about it is that I get to share it.

The other thing I just want to mention is I can't imagine having done this without my husband. It was such a fundamental experience, and we have been both working for this amount of time, creating pathways. If he had gone and done this, or I had gone and done it, without the other, it would have been a very different thing. Sharing this was a huge piece of it.

We all went on a trip together at the end of December, and it was the first time all of our blended family members had been together, other than at our wedding. I am going to chalk it up to our MDMA experience that I had never been, ever, ever, since the day my kids were born, more relaxed and present in the relationship. That was with six of them plus two boyfriends, not just my kids. I didn't want to be anywhere else. That's always been a challenge for me, is just being there. It was just fantastic. It wasn't conscious. It just happened.

On Saturday night, in a very impulsive moment, I texted J's ex-wife, and separately, my ex-husband's new wife, and said, "Hey, let's get together." And, of course, their reactions revealed their complete alarm. I woke up the next morning. I wasn't upset about it, but I just kind of laughed and went, "Wow, what the heck did I do that for?" I had two lovely, easy conversations that were just sort of a moment to say, "You know, it's all okay."

Then, I showed up Christmas with my ex-husband and his wife and my three kids. It's a situation that we have been trying to normalise for five years. It gets a little easier every year. This year, it was like nothing. I had a really good time. It's just so completely easy and wonderful. I didn't feel like I had to hold onto things to prove anything. I don't have this sense that my role is threatened if other people have some space at the table.

The other powerful experience that happened in-session was that I felt a real constriction in my throat. I just knew that it was about my voice. I've been trying to step into more of a leadership role and own the power that I think I have. I think part of that, texting the two women that I just described, was part of that. But it was also that I had felt seriously unleashed in my freedom to just say what is. It became not a big deal. I'm not talking about anything aggressive. I'm talking about it in a very productive way, and it just became so easy.

That's part of the gift that I want to share. There's a lot of strength that also feels really embedded. I think the organism, ourselves, when this does land, it's so grateful, it's going to take a lot to get it back to that earlier position, because it's allowed that to leave. Now, it's back to more who you really are, rather than who you are plus all the depredations and events that have happened during life.

S.'s comment in her final sentence is key: "Back to more who you really are" describes the essential trajectory of medicine work to allow us to engage with our psyches in such a way it can release us from many false beliefs. We may describe our lives as a journey along the lines of Pilgrim's Progress, but the truth of ourselves lies within us; as John Kabat-Zinn's book title states declaratively, 'Wherever You Go, There You Are.' This being the case, we do well when we open to our core selves, looking within to re-become the self of Tennyson who poetically describes our entry into the world: "Trailing Clouds of Glory Do We Come." This sweetest of events, our rebecoming, can only occur when we have come to peace with 'all the depredations' that have befallen us, leaving us in closer touch with who we really are.

Because of the many hours' distance between this couple and their attendant, it was not possible to have an in-person consultation before meeting for their first session. Communication devices with video are well and good and were utilised. This couple had bravely approached the work from recommendations of friends and their open-hearted, experiential descriptions of the work. This lack left S., 'definitely nervous' going into their first session, a condition that was ameliorated: 1) by her experience in that session, but also, 2) 'that fantastic conversation' we had immediately prior to their second session. This is tender, even intimate work, and the primary importance of trust underscores the incalculable value of having an in-person meeting with clients as they approach the work and before embarking on a session. The attendant's work is that of presence, and only by meeting together with clients prior to the session can that essential flesh-and-blood presence be established.

●   ●   ●

The first one was the big one.

Lex J.

Lex became interested in this work on behalf of his wife who had suffered severe trauma as a child. When she demurred, he was soon surprised to realise it was he who needed the work and made plans for himself. His first session turned things around for him in a major way, and he re-approached his wife whose attitude had still not changed. Until it did, and their work together went through many twists and turns as they both allowed the medicine to go deep and release their individual traumas.

I went to a book launch and began talking with a psychiatrist who spoke about this work, the Mithoefer study, and the success this work has had with severely treatment-resistant PTSD individuals, from which my wife had been suffering from PTSD for all the time I'd known her. I'm like, "Oh, my God, she needs to do this."

Then, I sat on it. My wife wasn't super into it. Then, there was a weekend that she went away. I was at home. I just couldn't settle, just crazy on the inside. I sat down and tried to meditate by the most beautiful river with the boats in the sunshine, and it was just hell on the inside. I was cycling back home when it suddenly hit me, "Oh, my God, I think *I* need to do this." I thought this was for her, but really, this is for me. I'd lost the number. I tried to contact the psychiatrist again. I saw that she was giving a talk and drove into the city, found her at this event, and asked her about meeting a facilitator. She said, "Well actually, you can talk to him right now."

When I was four, my parents divorced. My dad moved to Kenya, the other side of the world. That was one of my core traumas. In those days, we thought of therapists as bad things for sick people, not, "Hey, you know what, your son's life just changed, and maybe it would be good for him to have someone to talk to about it other than you." If I went to a psychiatrist, it would have been a sign that there was a problem. Stiff upper lip and all that. I didn't really think of it that way, because one never does. I was just me.

By the time I was twenty-two or something, the layers that I built on top of my trauma basically had me acting as an extroverted, outgoing, party guy who was into drugs, drinking ten cups of coffee a day and all over the place.

I had a health crisis when I was twenty-three. I went from being incredibly fit and able to take anything that I threw at myself to bedridden. For months, I was too exhausted to do more than walk down the end of the street. That was the start of material breaking through for me. On the surface, it manifested as a crisis in the physical, because I was not taking care of my physical body. The reason behind that was my anger and my abandonment issues, shame, fear of intimacy, and some considerable family trauma.

The only thing that made a difference for me was energy healing and complementary things, even though I didn't believe in them. It was a life-or-death thing. This was required to get me back at work. The toll that working took on me meant that I needed to keep going to see healers just to fill up the empty energy container. I got more stable maybe five or ten years into the process. This was not a curiosity thing; it was a necessity.

I went from bedridden to walking around. Nonetheless, fifteen years later, I was mostly functional but still had this underlying uneasiness with myself. So, I went to an MDMA facilitator and signed up for a first session with him.

I had taken psychedelics before and smoked pot, but the focus was more external than internal. I'd taken ayahuasca a couple of times and had deep internal experiences. I had several experiences in my own body that led me to suspect that I had experienced some violence as a child that I had blocked out—violence in the hands of my grandfather. I wasn't quite sure what was going on, but I had some flashes. I had a couple of experiences that deeply connected me to anger and my relationship to men and my fear of violence from men and that kind of thing.

It had come up in my body.

I was aware that I had a gap in my memory around a certain age. I had a reaction to men who were physically like my grandfather. When I was around violence, I'd shrink and pull back. I was just putting those clues together.

I thought, "Wow. There is a part of me I don't have access to. What's behind that?" It was clear that there was a tonne of shame behind it. These things, plus a life of searching and seeking—like a ten-day *vipassana* retreat that had been amazing—but still, I couldn't access something. That's what led me to go.

I was working now in the most intense environment I had ever worked in, at a senior position at a hedge fund, which is a very, very emotionally intense culture where your entire being is laid on the table for examination. I needed some support in that.

Was I nervous about taking the medicine? There is a level in me that is incredibly open, sensitive, and nervous all the time. Then, there is a place where I'm incredibly gung-ho, and I'd jump out of a helicopter. I think both of them were probably at play. My attendant had a really good way of helping me feel safe.

I went into it wanting to find out about my granddad and what was going on there. I lay on the couch with a blindfold on. It was a hot day, and the window was open. There was a bouncy castle in the street outside and a fair, and noises of children bubbled up through the window. That damn fan turned slowly. I started to drop and to drift. I remember my mind resting on my grandfather and just following some of his life. Just so much life and also so much trauma. In the session, I drifted along and experienced his story and then my grandparents and my mother. I felt this whole lineage history. That was in the more drifty part of the session. Then, some things got more intense, and this revelation about my life and things came through:

I'm lying in a boat. It's like a gondola, or a narrow wooden boat. I can see and feel the world on the inside of me. My attendant is in the back of the boat, and he is paddling. This is the River Styx. He is taking me across to the land of the dead. I'm dead in this boat. Then, the boat pulls up on the other side. I get up and get out of the boat. The boat moves away. I'm on my own.

Here I am, standing on the bank of the river. I look up. There is a wall stretching from horizon to horizon. Imagine the wall that was around the Secret Garden, but bigger. It's Victorian and faded, forbidding like stone but organic at the same time. I walk along the wall. I find a wrought-iron gate with a lot of stuff growing in it. It won't open. Then, blindfold off, I sit up, and I'm like, "Hey, can we talk for a minute? This happened. I'm here. I'm next to a wall. I think this may be the wall that I've been trying to get inside in me that has the shame and the trauma behind it. I can't get through. What do you recommend?"

My attendant says, "Talk to the wall." Gah! I put the blindfold on and lie back down.

The answer I get back is, "You don't have authority." I'm like, this is happening inside my mind. What do you mean I'm not allowed in?" It was very clear. "You don't have clearance to be in here." I'm the one who is telling me. I'm like, "What the fuck? I came here to get here. Now, there is no entry?"

Suddenly, my literal experience was that half the sky was light and heaven and had angels singing in it and represented all that was good. Half of the sky was the abyss and the total destruction of everything. It was only my attention to that line that was keeping everything from being swallowed by the abyss, all of reality.

I said, "I'm not entirely okay. I'm not entirely okay. Would you come and hold me?" He came, and he held me. I needed a lot of convincing that things were okay or were ever going to be okay in that place. In that moment, it was so real that I was in the flux of the universe. He gave me a grounded perspective; I remembered I was just a person having a traumatic experience, remembering the past. He held me and told me it would be okay. I made it. I wouldn't say that was some terrific victory or suddenly the sky had opened and the angels came and everything was great. No, but with his love and with his holding, I found my way. I got through.

Everything shifted. My experience with meditation shifted. My experience of sex shifted. My experience of human relationship shifted. That whole structure I'd been unwinding for my whole adult life fundamentally shifted that day. I mean the kind of thing that causes us to close off from seeing a piece of reality, just in order to get the daily things done.

I did more sessions. That's when I encountered my grandfather. I remember sitting next to him, some trauma thing being triggered, and him being violent to me in an unexplained way. Given that he was my hero after my father had left, this cracked something open. It feels like his trauma landed in my field. Trauma gets carried through generations and from perpetrators to victims and shapes the interpersonal and archetypal space.

I only had to visit the hell once. I wasn't actually in hell, but the fear itself very quickly becomes hell. I worked with that and the edge of fear again and again.

I started doing this work in 2003. My wife also started doing the work. On the one hand, that was amazing, because it freed a bunch of stuff up. On the other hand, we had a marriage that was an uneasy vehicle for carrying our traumas. Although the

MDMA shifted some things that allowed us to be more present and intimate with each other, and although we'd been working together on the inner space for eight years and been through all kinds of healing, shit started to get brought up for both of us that basically led our marriage to blow up within six months of us both starting to do the work.

I left the marriage. Three months later, divorce papers were filed. We were trying to have a conversation about assets, but we just couldn't talk. I wrote to her and said, "Look, it would just be really shitty if we never spoke again and had to do the rest of this through lawyers. I don't care what it takes. You name what situation, what circumstances." I gave a list of options. One of which was, "We could go take MDMA together." I had wanted to do MDMA with her as my last grasp thing for trying to fix what was going on.

She said no. Three months later, she emailed me back and said yes. We had this extraordinary experience, because we had been time-sharing the house. We were both looking after the house and the cats but swapping over at different times, never seeing each other. We were doing the dance that we do when we're pretending to be separate beings.

Still, we showed up for the session. It was awkward. We went to separate couches, and we took our medicine, and we lay down. This experience of being ten feet away, of being aware of her process but not in her process, having everything about her prime in my mind so that she is in my whole process as this beautifully separate being doing her own work on the other side of the room, was magically healing.

That's how this work works for couples. I had my own journey. She had her own journey. When we came together, we were very open. I was still very clearly done with the marriage, but then we started talking and found out that the couples' therapist we had both been seeing had been giving us incompatible advice and seemed to have had an agenda for trying to separate us.

Everyone has their part to play in the divine play. It was six months before we were back together, but that turned the supertanker around. I don't know if MDMA saved our marriage, because maybe it's destined and something else would have happened, but if it wasn't the work, it was going to have to be something really big. Without the work, I don't think we would be where we are now.

The foundation of my marriage came back together. I treat this work as extremely sacred. I treat people involved in this work as family.

This is such valuable work.

Working with Lex and his wife over a number of sessions, it became clear that their love for each other was both sincere and intact; they laughed and smiled and finished each other's sentences and so on. Over time, the image I had of them drew from Tim O'Brien's 1990 book, "The Things They Carried," that described the burdensome equipment that foot soldiers in Vietnam, the grunts, were required to carry on their backs into battle. Similarly, it was as if these two each entered their marriage in love with each other but with a huge backpack of traumatic material, each of which began to spew their contents upon them in a toxic mix as they did their level best for ten years to live as man and wife. The work with MDMA enabled them to put much of their burden down, to reframe their relationship with each other and resume their love story.

• • •

CHAPTER FOUR

The Healing Trajectory

———

"You gain strength, courage and confidence by every experience in which you really stop to look fear in the face. You are able to say to yourself, 'I have lived through this horror. I can take the next thing that comes along.' You must do the thing you think you cannot do."

ELEANOR ROOSEVELT

MDMA enables an enormous expansion of consciousness. Clients are so engulfed in what is going on within them, they may not talk to their attendant at all. There may be interactions and conversations, but back-and-forth conversation is always kept to a necessary minimum; words are more of a footnote to what's going on inside. In addition, our vocabulary of spoken words is a tool in ordinary consciousness, but once MDMA takes effect, and we're talking to someone in a non-ordinary state from our ordinary state, any conversation may inadvertently be at cross-purposes, limiting comprehension.

If a client has concerns, or they want to talk, of course, that's fine. We respond to their needs, but we remain essentially outside their experience. The important thing is that it is the client who is moved to talk, not the attendant. An attendant who talks too much or tries to guide the session with verbal prompts is behaving in a way that is not only irrelevant to the client's inner journey, but risks derailing the trajectory of the session itself, which occurs entirely within the client.

The attendant's role is supportive, not prescriptive. In one session, for instance, the client wanted to chat. She sat on the edge of the couch, talking non-stop for fifteen to twenty minutes. The attendant let her go on, listened for a pause, and then gently asked her if she would like to put on the eyeshades and lie down. She said, "Oh!" and looked around. While she was chatting, she had completely forgotten why she was there.

She put on the eyeshades and lay back on the couch where she stayed for the next four hours. She lay as still as a log, in utter silence, experiencing whatever came up. This woman led a very public life and had come to work with MDMA to address an occupational hazard, the easy availability of alcohol at the many events she attended. After that session, she stopped drinking.

Clients understand that the attendant has no plan for how the session will run. They need only to trust, surrender and receive the medicine, allowing it to approach them and to engage with whatever it reveals.

With MDMA, the cognitive processing function is still in action, but it becomes secondary to the feeling experience. Our thinking brain is usually dominant, essential for the planning and organising we need to achieve in our lives. Under the medicine, the executive functioning part of our brain steps back a bit and makes room for an inundation of information from our somatic, feeling capacity.

Although we may not ordinarily think of emotions as carriers of information, they most certainly are. Feelings are a repository of information from every area of our lives, and flooding the brain with serotonin lets us access the archives of our subconscious in a new, uninhibited way. Cognitive processing may help us integrate these feelings down the road, but during the session, we are free to focus on the feelings that emerge. Cognitive function, while still clear and bright, becomes secondary.

We also tend to see feelings as problematic, even dangerous. We assume our emotional states need managing, directing, and corralling. Extreme emotions worry many of us; what if we feel murderous, suicidal, or psychotic? We're afraid of where our emotions might take us. Pharmaceutical drugs are designed to manage that fear by suppressing such extreme feelings. By contrast, by trusting in the process during a medicine session, we can fully engage with whatever feelings come up. The client has nothing to do, literally, but surrender to the medicine as it approaches and immerse her- or himself in the feelings as they arise.

NO WORDS CAN SAY

"The psychiatrist who has not studied the bio-energetic functions of the emotions is apt to overlook the organism as such and to remain stuck in the psychology of words and associations."

WILHELM REICH, M. D.

In the orthodox therapist-client relationship, words are the coin of the realm. The therapist and the client talk together about issues brought into the therapy room by the client; about family issues, about their parents, siblings and other actors, their fears, indeed about anything that the client wants to bring up in the session. Everything is on the table. The therapist responds with thoughts about whatever issues have been raised, giving advice and recommendations per their training, and the therapeutic conversation continues.

In this medicine work, we may talk about this and that before and after the session, but during it, the client is so engaged with what is being revealed within themselves that talk is adjunctive only. The need to talk *about* our mother is radically supplanted by our newfound ability to talk *with* our mother as she becomes graphically experienced, revivified and utterly present under the medicine's influence. The mother is not a simple memory evoked by our cognitive attention and focus. She is presented unbidden by the psyche, without evocation by us, as being the most important thing for us to look at. She is psychically present to us just as she was physically present to us. The client has nothing to do but allow.

"Tell me and I will forget. Show me and I will remember. Involve me and I will understand."

LAO TZU

This in-session ability results from the non-ordinary consciousness occasioned by the medicine allowing the frozen present, the captured memory from the past, to arrive into the present moment. The psyche realises that the personal circumstances it had captured and has been holding onto have another timeframe: Now.

The psyche comes to understand that there is considerable time and space between the tumult of the past and the peacefulness of the present. It understands in present time that the terrible emotional event is over and done with, that the client is now safe, and the threat is past. With this new understanding, the psyche reverses itself and releases its hold on the traumatic memories it had originally captured.

RELEASING TRAUMA

"Since feeling is first, he who pays any attention to the syntax of things will never wholly kiss you..."

E. E. CUMMINGS

Dr. Bessel van der Kolk, a leading trauma specialist in the US, writes about the importance of focusing on the bodily and emotional experience in his paradigm-shifting book, *The Body Keeps the Score.* He writes about the essential flaw he sees in conventional therapy, talking about something when it should be felt. When Dr. van der Kolk was becoming a psychiatrist, he went through his own analysis and became frustrated trying to explain his feelings to his analyst. As soon as he started using words, it became a cognitive process rather than a direct experience. The feeling was gone.

Trauma takes a tremendous toll on human energy. Much of our energy is dedicated to maintaining our distance from the trauma held within, to keep it from popping up in our lives as troublesome symptoms and affecting our behaviour. That energy is *our* energy; our life force that eventually becomes exhausted by protecting us from our traumatic memories, leaving us with no remaining energy to enjoy life. The organism comes to understand the hopelessness of the double-bind it is in, a situation that can only result in exhaustion and depression.

MDMA works directly and synergistically with the body's physiological and emotional responses with no middle man needed. Because of this intense, personal, and intimate level of processing, the changes brought about by the medicine are not only profound at the moment they emerge, they are permanent. The medicine's power, remarkably, lasts long beyond the session itself; what is released in a session stays released. There may be more traces of trauma still to be released in a future session, but what is gone is gone.

The staying power can be attributed to the way MDMA works with the body's own physiology. The trauma was captured by the psyche at the height of the traumatic event and subsequently maintained within us as an inchoate memory. Once it is released, the psyche has no possible motive to recapture it, and we are open to the possibility it is as pleased to see the back of it as we, ourselves, are. We are, after all, indivisible.

Other compassionate practices follow the same biological logic. Dr. van der Kolk recommends methods like EMDR and yoga, that also help traumatised people feel comfortable enough within themselves to allow the traumatic material to rise and release. MDMA therapy is in accord with this understanding, utilising the body's own innate healing capabilities to create permanent change.

Although the healing that occurs on the day of the medicine session is remarkable, it's always part of a journey that starts long before the client ever knocks on our door. The trajectory of healing includes everything the person has done before, how they came to the work, why they came to the work, how they feel about it, and how it affects their life in the future.

Most clients have tried many therapeutic "cures" but finding their condition is treatment-resistant, they decide to try MDMA. Everybody has experienced therapy, which may have been helpful but was ultimately an incomplete solution to their problems. A high percentage of individuals have been prescribed psychopharmacological agents in the past. One client who came to us said he had been on every medication made by the pharmaceutical industry for over ten years. He was given Prozac after an episode of anxiety and depression at college, and mixes of dozens of other drugs since then. One doctor would say, "Take drugs ABC," and the next would say, "Try drugs XYZ." Literally. Not only did none of these medications help, but many of them made things worse. This young man was a superstar at the London School of Economics, but he was not able to maintain even a basic level of functioning while taking antidepressants. His career trajectory tanked.

He grew up in a large Jewish family, but was essentially alone in his adult life. Estranged from his mother, father, and brother, he lived alone in a single room. The client had been so depressed for so long, he couldn't imagine not being depressed. Yet, after the first session, speaking from his familiarity with psychopharmaceutical drugs, he said that MDMA does for depression what Ativan does for anxiety. "An hour and a half in," he said, "I wasn't depressed. For the first time in over ten years, I did not feel depressed."

Relieving acute depression is reason enough to consider MDMA, but clients also go on to do mindful work outside of the session that contributes to their healing. When this client got his functioning back, and he could finally talk with his father, he asked if he remembered anything particularly noteworthy from his infancy. His father said, "Oh, my God, you were the clingiest child! We could not put you down. You had to be with us all the time. We had to sleep with you."

With this perspective, he could see that having an anxiety attack in college, the first time he was separated from his mother, may have triggered the stress of separation he felt as an infant. The intensity of these feelings took him to the college psychiatrist; it was not an isolated incident but attached to his childhood biographical development.

An interesting question here is how things might have turned out if the childhood anxiety had been treated differently. If he had been handled in such a way as a baby that did not result in anxiety, would the outcome have been different for the adult? It is impossible to say, but one can imagine that this man might have been spared depressive episodes, anxiety attacks, and over ten years of psychiatric drugs.

This client, even with all those years of missed opportunities, is now functioning well. He has a girlfriend and meaningful work. He loves and is engaged with his family, who are wholeheartedly on his side. His life has been turned around in a very good way.

SUPPRESS OR EXPRESS?

The action of MDMA is to open us up, resulting in our willing and courageous exposure to experience the dark psychic material that has been misguiding our lives and to encourage its expression. The action of pharmaceutical drugs is to shut us down, suppressing our ability to feel, which effectively closes us off from the possibility of finding release. We need to know and experience what it is that needs to be released, before the psyche can release it.

For those who do access the psychiatric system of prescription drugs, the benefit is dubious. Too many spend years spinning their wheels, trying different preparations but getting no closer to the source of the dysfunction. Going on and coming off antidepressants can be traumatising, and clients approaching work with MDMA must declare their prescription drug use before any sessions can be undertaken. They may or may not be problematic, but the class of drugs called psychoactives, SSRI's in particular, most definitely are, requiring the client to taper down and then wait six weeks to allow for the psychopharmacological drug to completely exit the body. Working with skilled psychopharmacologists, we help clients navigate certain antidepressants and any other agents that are incompatible with MDMA treatment. The express action of MDMA comes into direct conflict with the suppress action of psychopharmacological agents, which then work against each other.

AFTERCARE

The experience with the medicine is both profound and information-rich, and clients continue to work with the material that has been unearthed long after the session. This integration may come through formal psychotherapy sessions that seek to ground the in-session experiences with consensus reality. The integration may be essential if we are to be able to maintain the benefit from the insights and epiphanies gained. This approach may be described as "psychotherapy-assisted MDMA."

However, our clients have found, almost universally, meditation is a logical extension of their MDMA session as well as a very effective way to integrate the insights they have gained. Integration can also result from insights reached in normal conversations with friends, family, and interested colleagues, underscoring the importance of allowing sufficient time between sessions for such events to occur. Inquiring of clients about their outside support group is key to ensure they gain maximum benefit from the medicine. They need to have a psychotherapist, a meditation practice, a best friend, or a yoga group with whom they can engage. Talking about things may not be part of the process during the active medicine work, but it is essential in ordinary consciousness to understand and integrate the material that has emerged during this important, potentially watershed moment in their lives.

An analogous situation may be found with commonly established protocols around surgery. The operating theatre is sacrosanct, and post-op the patient enters the Intensive Care Unit (ICU) for aftercare. Similarly, the medicine session room is sacrosanct, and post-session, the client enters what we might also call the ICU; Integration and Continued Understanding.

SHARING

Many clients, at the conclusion of a session, are eager to recommend the medicine to someone else they know. People have said, "I wish I had known about this. My friend committed suicide from Iraq," or, "My brother needs this." Almost everybody knows somebody they think could benefit from this work.

The impulse, of course, is to go right out and proselytise, but we strenuously advise clients not to try to persuade others to expose themselves to MDMA. The best way for them to share their experience is to live an engaged post-MDMA life and trust that people will see the change and might remark, "Hey, you seem very relaxed." With such an opening, the client can follow their lead and start a conversation about the work that can inform them and enable them to make their own decision about getting involved.

We often see several clients from the same family. We insist that each client approach us personally and take responsibility for their own involvement, absent any input from their referee. If a client thinks his cousin might be interested, we ask, "Please have your cousin send us an e-mail." In this way, the potential client's interest is assuredly their own, and each individual is taking responsibility for their own situation and doing whatever they, themselves, need to do to address it.

And it felt like it was just more me.

A.D.A.

At thirty-five years of age, the incoherence of A.D.A.'s presentation at our initial consultation was both problematic and revealing. He was a highly creative, intelligent, and sensitive child who experienced generational, systemic, and family trauma. including a painful divorce and years spent living with an 'alcoholic and abusive' stepfather. This unresolved past contributed to a series of failed relationships which left him feeling hopeless and suicidal.

The first session released him from any wish to take his own life, and three subsequent sessions made the causal factors of his multifaceted dysfunction sufficiently coherent that his therapist felt he 'had accomplished the goals he had set for therapy.' The following testimony is of a conversation between A.D.A., his somatic therapist and the attendant (A.).

When I was eighteen, I had an experience of being given messages that led me to believe that, with enough faith, I could teleport

500 miles to visit my girlfriend. This attempt would be accomplished by driving my VW Fox into the back of an eighteen-wheel semi on I-79.

I was shocked to find myself on the side of the road, face-to-face with an angry truck driver. I simply told the state police the truth. They called my parents, and my mother took me to see a psychiatrist. I didn't trust his prescription of antipsychotics as the answer. To protect myself, I basically just stopped talking about what I was experiencing and feeling for the next decade or so.

At thirty-two, after a string of back-and-forth breakups with a woman in San Francisco, I found myself suicidal on the Golden Gate Bridge. Out of desperation, I decided to meet with a psychiatrist, and she diagnosed me with bipolar. The past decade had been filled with deep depressions, manic visions, and uncontrolled productivity as well as crashes and experiences of interacting directly with both Jesus Christ and Lucifer, and so the description of the symptoms seemed to fit. I was, however, deeply sceptical of Western psychiatry's ability to provide any sort of true healing.

Early on, my psychiatrist asked me what my relationship was to emotion. I said, "Well, I don't see any point in having negative emotions." And that really was who I had become. There was this part of me that was spending so much energy just keeping anything that was difficult to face at bay.

Eventually, she put me on a little lithium, and I noticed it was basically doing the same thing—holding back difficult emotions. It was reinforcing this ego structure that was trying to keep emotions away. It felt like putting mortar on a brick wall that

I really needed to come down. So, I made a conscious decision one day to secretly go off the medicine and to feel whatever was beneath the surface.

I didn't have any guidance, but I had a vision. I was in my bed and literally, a shimmering green woman appeared at my side and in her outstretched palms she offered me my pain as medicine. So, I drank it, and I went into myself and confronted an ice cold, writhing ball of black eels. They engulfed me, and I spent four hours on that bed just convulsing. I thought I was going to die; I felt like I died. I passed out, and when I woke up, I had such a sense of calm and peace and just this voice that said, "Kindness goes a long way."

That experience convinced me of the importance of my emotions, but I'd quickly find out I was far from finished. A lifetime of avoiding my *self* had saddled me with relational patterns that would soon bring me to the edge once more, deeply broken, and suicidal.

By the time of his consultation with the medicine work attendant, he was experiencing 'a perfect storm' precipitated by another series of breakups and a sense of complete hopelessness of ever being in a loving relationship. He spoke of a prior diagnosis of schizophrenia and bipolar, of anxiety, paranoia, and depression, and that he was 'really suicidal.'

One medicine session was conducted:

Going in, I was terrified of all sorts of things. That I'd go insane. That I'd be damned to hell. But I also sensed this could help me access, feel, and heal more deeply than I was able to do on my own and that this was my last choice. I had told myself that I'd try this, and if it didn't work, I'd kill myself.

From behind the darkness of my eye mask arose a topography of the major traumas of my life. I saw on the horizon three mountains: My parents' divorce at age eight; the death of a girlfriend's father at eighteen; and a devastating romantic relationship at thirty-two. In addition, there was a gentle, wise, and guiding voice asking me, "Would you like to look at this? Are you ready?"

"Yes," I said. Over the next couple hours, I would hold each event from multiple angles. Turning them over and over until one by one, each of them simply blew away like sand, and in its place a deeper sense of relaxation and acceptance.

In the same way I was guided and saw these major events release and disappear, this inner voice appeared, and I saw that this wasn't the medicine talking—it was me. That I had the capacity to be kind and loving and wise. That I was lovable and capable of loving. And it felt like it was just more me.

After that first session, I went from having what I've described as an Encyclopedia Britannica of negative self-talk to almost nothing, like a Tweet, overnight. Once in a while, a whisper of a sentence creeps in, but it was just gone, never to return after that session.

When explaining to a friend online my experience of relating to myself, they suggested that I check out somatic therapy.

I looked into it thought, "Man, they're teaching therapists to be with their patients the way I was with myself at the peak of this

MDMA experience, and that's fascinating." The self I want to integrate, it's like they gave someone a guidebook of how to be that with their patients and that oriented me to say, "Go find someone because you'll have a person who is modelling relating to you in the way that you want to relate to yourself."

From this beginning, he found a somatic therapist, who shared:

"In my work, I invite the client into an active process of inquiry to their relational and survival style. Although there are seemingly endless emotional challenges, I believe they all derive from early trauma which impairs the connection to self and others. So, in the sessions, the client reflects on their own internal process, and we explore how (and why) the client creates their own perpetuating symptoms—to help them recognise their agency. In essence, we explore what's coming in the way of their connection, attunement, trust, autonomy, or love for themselves and others.

"It's a unique approach, because it combines somatically oriented psychoanalytically informed therapy, which includes identity, personality, and how it plays out in relationships. In other words, what are their difficulties in their way of connecting with others? And a lot will come up—a lot of shame and a lot of pride-based identification.

"A.D.A. came to see me with two goals in mind: First, he wanted to process and integrate some unresolved developmental trauma, which he felt would help him be more present, and second, he wanted to have a successful, healthy relationship. He described his history as follows: Diagnosis of schizophrenia at eighteen, which was later changed to bipolar as he had bouts of mania and depression. Contrary to the psychiatrist's recommendation for pharmacological interventions, he decided not to take the medications and to interpret the diagnosis as 'dharma rather that dogma.' He planned to explore other ways of working with his emotional extremes.

"He told me that prior to our meeting, he had taken MDMA therapeutically, which he stated had the effect of 'stopping all his negative self-talk.' The medicine had also brought to the surface a memory of an isolated event in which his uncle may have molested him. At our meetings, initially intermittent, then weekly, A. shared instances which revealed some paranoia, i.e., his roommate was an undercover agent who had formulated a plot against him and was going to report him to the authorities for using MDMA, or that satanic or dark fears were obsessing him, making him feel a bit out-of-control, or that I was really a witch. In all the sessions, we explored his subjective, somatic responses, his internal processing, his emotions, and his relationship with (E), his partner."

During a subsequent medicine session, A. addressed the possibility that his uncle had molested him.

For a few years, I had this confusion around if my uncle, who had been a known paedophile, had, in fact, molested me in some way. I had wrestled with somatic symptoms and a fuzzy memory of being alone with him in his van. During my third medicine session, I was determined to go into the confusion and figure out what happened, and so I did. As if emerging from underwater to take a breath, I came back with a puzzling feeling—that perhaps this memory was of a doctor putting a thermometer in my butt as a baby, and it had become conflated with the fear we all had of this uncle growing up. There was such a sense of relief and release with this and also a feeling that no matter what happened, it didn't really matter anymore. Molestation or doctor, whatever it was I had been obsessing about, just went away.

I spoke with my parents about this recent medicine experience, and my mother said, "You know what, A.? There was something that happened that I hadn't even realised happened to you." She said that when I was really young, five weeks or six weeks old, I was having a difficult time going. I was constipated, and so she took me to this doctor that she had never taken me to before, and his solution was to put a rubber glove on and just stick his finger in my ass to loosen it up. She said, "I was horrified. I was like what the hell? You started crying, and this whole thing, and he said, 'Oh, we're just gonna loosen some things up in there, stretch his anus out so he can go to the bathroom better.'"

As she told this story, it felt in my body like that was actually what had happened. That this was an old somatic experience that I was trying to make sense of and that the experience of being terrified of this uncle seemed like a possible explanation.

I was like, "That seems to be actually even a more accurate experience that could have happened." It seems to me like that could have just as easily been the core thing that happened somatically, but I didn't have a story around it. But I also did have this uncle that had molested kids and who we were terrified of, and there was this story, this memory of something in the van, and people being afraid. "Don't go near the uncle," and this whole thing.

This medicine, it really helps heal the shame that we pick up along our lives. For example, there was a period of about a year between my first and second session, where I was really paranoid and interacting with some deeply archetypal stuff.

The suicidal thoughts and negative self-talk were gone, but I was still very afraid and ashamed. I heard the voice of a very angry Jesus condemning me, and I came face-to-face with demons and confronted the devil.

In addition, there was this general fear and paranoia about people close to me. I thought that the two of you (therapist and medicine-attendant) were a witch and warlock secretly in cahoots to steal my soul.

But the interesting thing was, after I unwound the anxiety and paranoia (which happened almost immediately in the second session), I was able to see, "Oh, these are people that care about you." And this part of yourself that felt unlovable, I needed to kind of create a story that they must be up to something; they certainly are not here just for me. The speed of release was fascinating. During that second session, I confronted the paranoia and anxiety directly. I saw it for what it was. I laughed at it and understood on a deep level that this is never going to be here again. There's no more need for it. It just went, "Whoosh!"

A.: It had already been released?

Yes! In that moment, whatever was generating that paranoia and anxiety, *it* was just gone. I was more clearly able to experience the separation and distinction between who I was and whatever these adaptive responses of which I was letting go.

His therapist observed:

"Your experience moved from an 'I' to an 'it', and you were removed from your experience. Initially, your paranoia was part of you and gradually through your work, the paranoia was something you experienced, and you were removed from it.

"Simultaneous with our work, A. did one session with mushrooms, which he described as a sacred experience, and an additional two or three more guided sessions with MDMA, which he referred to as medicine. He shared that the attendant sat with him, and he went deep inside and felt the medicine was engaging with him and helping him gain new insights about his past as well as his relationship with his partner. What struck me was the incredible metamorphosis I witnessed.

"As time progressed, it was evident to me that A.D.A had transformed his entire being, his way of organising his *self*, his identity, and his thoughts. Even more, the way he carried himself started to change. What he wanted to address in therapy was changing; there were no longer any bouts of paranoia or disordered thinking. In February, he stated that he no longer felt any depression, that he only felt anxious at times, and that he is able to hold the feeling and himself with compassion as he feels the anxiety. He explored and physiologically integrated the instance of abuse by his uncle. He had accomplished his goals that he had set for therapy—that of greater presence and a deep connection and emotionally engaging relationship with E. As such, we decided to end his therapy with the understanding that if he wants to explore more, he will return at a different time in the future."

Following his first medicine session, A.D.A. had found the perfect situation to discuss his experiences with a somatic trauma therapist, and as she skillfully objectified his paranoia, he came to understand the reality or unreality of his inner voices. He heard them, but finally knew they were not him. The medicine work is interactive within the session, requiring our finest attention, and it also needs to be interactive without the session. We cannot do this work alone, and after he had returned to ordinary consciousness following his medicine work, he found sense and reason by engaging with a therapist who teased his paranoid feelings apart.

A.D.A. had come by one evening after meeting with her and said she had 'fired' him, and my delight at this outcome only mirrored his own.

A.D.A. had been actively involved with the elements of his inner life since his teenage years. His observation of the mechanism-of-action of lithium being but one example, and another of his observations deserves some unpacking. In the second paragraph, he says, "There was this part of me that was spending so much energy just keeping anything that was difficult at bay." The trauma that has been caught and held within us requires, unbeknownst to us, our fierce attention every hour of the day to manage and contain. It is this endeavour, described since psychology's infancy as 'anger turned inwards,' that consumes our life force, our élan vital, our prana, our chi to the point where literally no energy remains for life itself. The organism comes to understand that the physical, psychic, and spiritual exhaustion it is experiencing cannot be resolved and there is no way forward. We are spent. This is the very definition of depression.

• • •

I think it's good to keep in mind that emotion is also information.

Charley W.

We are adamant that all individuals entering the work with MDMA have support systems that may include spiritual disciplines, yoga, meditation, psychotherapy, and other therapeutic modalities to help with integration of the material that arises in the medicine sessions. Our method of operation is to maintain the treatment room as a sacred space, inviolable to any influence from theories emanating from outside, whether religious, philosophical, psychotherapeutic, or psychiatric. With the room free from uninvited intervention and clear of any influence whatsoever, the client surrenders to the creation of the non-ordinary consciousness that permits the psyche to open, precipitating release from the toxic material it has caught and held throughout their lives. Following the session, when the client is returned to ordinary consciousness, many disciplines can be used as invaluable tools for integration. Here, a psychotherapist shares his approach to working with individuals following their medicine sessions.

People who use the medicine are generally the type of people who are into self-awareness, self-growth, and exploration. They are the type of people who make the best kind of therapy patient, because they're ripe and ready for growth. It's a self-selective process. The type of person who is doing the medicine work is generally an explorer and serious about their own personal growth, and is using the medicine as a catalyst.

For the person who undertakes a medicine session and comes to me afterwards, the question hanging in the air is, "How do I live this? I just had this amazing experience," perhaps one that has been either wonderful or difficult or both, but certainly deep. "How do I get this into my life? How do I integrate this?"

Sometimes a session with medicine involves opening deep, hidden, or traumatic material that had not been available to them. Then, they can come in and work on these things piece by piece. For example, I've had one person come in who had had one session with the medicine and was in therapy with me for about six to seven months just to integrate everything that came up during that one session.

So much gets stirred up or exposed and kicked up. Sometimes, it's disturbing. Sometimes, it's a revelation. They want to integrate that into their lives in a way that's going to work. The emotional expansion the medicine allows is so huge! Also, I think often we forget that emotion is also information. This information needs to be processed.

It's never a good idea to suppress a feeling. That doesn't mean you must act on every feeling, of course. If you're angry, that doesn't mean you act on the anger every time. But it's information. Often, anger means you've been violated in some way by somebody, or you perceive that you have, or you think that you have. The anger, in such a case, is your reaction against it. Therefore, your anger is important information about what's happening to or around you.

I welcome people who have taken medicine and treat them just as I would any other client, but often with an extra degree of respect.

Sometimes, it is surprising and disturbing for them. My job is to help them befriend their material, turn what could feel like a demon into an ally. The important thing is that some people think the medicine is an end unto itself, and for some people it is, but usually it kicks up stuff that just starts the process. Then, the work is to really go into the depth of that material, so that one can make it a part of their life and find strength from it.

There are some techniques that I use for integrating. One is writing about the medicine session, about the time with the medicine, as a way of just getting it further into your bones. When they write about it, then they can bring it into a therapy session.

There's also an anchoring technique which I and others have found to be useful. When I have used the medicine, for example, I may make a point of being aware of that very warm, expansive, loving, and safe feeling in my chest. Then, afterward, I can recall this sensation physically, and this can remind me of that safe feeling and that feeling of well-being. I can carry it with me. So, if the person has experienced the medicine within the last couple of days or so, I will help them recall and get back in touch with the experience in a physical way, thereby anchoring it into their being.

Another such technique is with music. I know someone who listened to an Enya piece in a medicine session called, "Flora's Secret," which is just a lovely song. Afterwards, if she had had a stressful day at work, driving home in the car, she could play this song and that feeling of serenity would return.

Then, there are ways I use to help people integrate material in the session using Gestalt techniques. I'm trained in Gestalt Therapy. So, if there's somebody in your life that hurt you or angered you, I have you imagine they're in a chair and you're facing them in your chair and talking to them as if they were right there in the room. That can be a very powerful technique.

Sometimes, if somebody says, reminiscing, "My mother never held me," or, "My mother never picked me up," or anything like that, I say, "Can you say it to your mother?" And they say, "Mommy, you never held me." The depth of feeling becomes totally different, because then they're engaged in the present moment.

Another thing I like to do with clients is teach them mindfulness techniques. I have found that working with the medicine, for myself, gets me into that state where my mind quiets down, my thoughts quiet down and slow down, and I'm in a place where I'm more present and more rooted in the moment and mindful of everything around me. I find that mindfulness meditation is a useful way of integrating the experience into my life.

I have been impressed by the mindfulness people exhibit. After a medicine session, they have noticed things they have never noticed before and have sometimes changed their behaviour toward other people, like not reacting out of anger. In terms of personal growth, the beginning of consciousness is to become really mindful of what we are doing. This can occur when we're making a cup of tea or running a business meeting.

I realise that in terms of my own growth, I sometimes lack mindfulness in a therapy session. I have fear about letting the session go wherever it's going to go. I tell myself sometimes, they're paying me good money, so if there's silence, and they're looking to me for an answer, and if I don't fill in the time, and I don't make something happen, they're going to think I'm stupid or incompetent, or they're wasting their time and money. So, then, I might try to make something happen. Sometimes, that works, but often it just doesn't. I would like to learn how to be more about letting go of the whole process and letting things just evolve organically and trust that the session can develop in a natural way.

The urge to 'try to make something happen' that this therapist references in his final paragraph is legitimate within the context of an inter-psychic talk therapy session. For our work as attendants, awareness of this urge is part of our thinking as we endeavour to protect the client from any outside influence during the session, particularly psychiatric and psychological constructs. While under the influence of MDMA, we are more suggestible than in ordinary consciousness, so even well-meaning suggestions made with the best of intentions can intrude on the inner workings of the client, potentially derailing the psychic information they are engaging within themselves. For this reason, we have found that contemplatives, meditators who welcome not only a few hours of silence but also the opportunity to be in service, are the ideal attendants for this work.

I would like to acknowledge this therapist's clear identification of feelings as information. We normally think of information as facts known to us or presented to us, but we trash our entire feeling capacity if we discount their nature as carriers of information. Vital information, as it turns out.

• • •

And I was just having these awful panic attacks.

Elijah S.

Elijah's single session was revelatory to him, and he knew right away that he had a lot to talk about with the person who referred him to the work, Walter, his clinical psychologist of many years standing. He was eager, arriving for his medicine session before the appointed time. By 11:00 a.m., he had taken the first dose of MDMA and was comfortably situated on the couch awaiting results. It was some time before he felt the effects of the medicine, but when he did, it was off to the races, and there he stayed and stayed and stayed, until taking a nap before leaving around 8:30 p.m. The following is an excerpt from a second follow-up session with his therapist, conducted around ten days after the medicine work session, at which his attendant, A., was also present. We get some flavour of the longstanding, close, and supportive relationship they had created and maintained—humorous, earthy, and real.

WALTER: With each person I talk to afterwards, they each have a different journey. Elijah was so clear, and I've been thinking about it, and I think I said it to you last time. Because you were a philosophy major, there was something already underway. Philosophy majors seem to take to it like a fish to water, because there's that something in the brain that already wants to go to strange places.

ELIJAH: Yeah. Well, the funny thing was I didn't think I would go to any…I mean, I'm very happy with where I went, but I didn't think I was going to go there. I thought I would work through the parents, the family, the self-confidence, self-hatred, whatever stuff that you work on in therapy for years and years. We've also worked together for quite a long time before this.

W: That's right.

E: I think that brought me an immense level of comfort to begin with, which gave me a lot of flexibility and a lot of tools, also. We had focused on moving one's mind around on being present in your surroundings, on the importance of exercise, and I feel that may have helped me just rip through everything so quickly and get on to bigger and brighter things, shall we say?

W: Yeah. Let's go to that. Talk about whatever you had in mind that you wanted to say today.

E: I guess in terms of what brought me to it, which was the initial question, I had been working with various therapists in one capacity or another for…Oh, geez. I think I was like six years old or something? Nothing really ever got better. It just changed and got worse, and got worse in new ways. Then, we met when I was in college, worked together for a year and a half maybe. I was a junior in college.

W: Right. It was on and off, sprinkled.

E: Sprinkled, certainly, which was very good, introducing me to things like Neurontin, which helped me sleep a lot at the time. That was very helpful. I would say it definitely suppressed the underlying issues to a point where things were good.

W: Why did it suppress it?

E: Well, I had someone really to talk about it with, you, that was able to provide other solutions rather than the very harmful drinking, fighting, basically, one form or another of self-abuse that I engaged in to relieve that tension. You provided other avenues for it.

W: Do you remember what the avenue was?

E: It was mostly moving one's mind. We've been doing a thing with books for many, many years.

W: You once said something, also, that had important meaning. That there was a father role, which I always discounted, because I'm not into all that. But it simplified therapy, because, if you think about it, if I could build enough relationship where I could have the simple father role, then all I have to do is give you advice in a supportive fatherly way and you're bound to listen to it, which is the kind of person you are.

E: Yeah, that's true.

W: Because if someone's loved and supported, then if the person who loves them and supports them says something, they're bound not to put up the biggest fight in the world.

E: Oh, no, that's a very good point. I forgot about the whole transference thing. Yeah, and we had a chuckle and said, "That's true." I believe, you said, "Yeah, that'll happen. Don't take it too seriously," and we moved on.

So, you know I left college and got to work at a job out of school at a very prominent law firm, which I thoroughly despised, and it sort of sent me right down the toilet in terms of the way I treated myself and the way I felt about the world. Breaking from that after a year, I moved to a role in real estate. I became rather obsessed with my own physical fitness and health. So, that was all right, but the job in itself sucked, and I had no emotional connection to it.

Then, unfortunately, or fortunately, depending on how you look at it in a grander scheme of the way things move, around last summer, things just began to fall, you know, all kinds of ways. My father became very, very ill. I moved from that job into a new job which turned out to be an absolute disaster. Didn't make it more than a few weeks. I had a girl who I was very, very close with, and we ended up splitting up.

And I was just having these awful panic attacks. Couldn't even think during them. Crippling. Couldn't drive. Truly, it was a nightmare. Absolute nightmare. Could barely do anything functional. So, that led me back here, actually. Credit to that girl, she said, "You have to call somebody now. I'm not leaving until you call somebody. You must know somebody. You have to call somebody."

So, that's how we ended up speaking again. Subsequently, after a few sessions, I was connected with a psychiatrist who gave me the diagnosis of Bipolar Two, so I've been using Lamictal since then, scaling it up to 200 milligrams a day which I take now, and that helped a lot.

w: Yes, it did.

E: That helped it a lot. And through our work, things really improved, you know. I ended up getting a phenomenal job at a company I've been interested in for years in September. The family situation, I came to deal with it much better.

w: Yes. Very well.

E: Much better through our work and that was really...

w: To your credit.

E: Well, to your credit as well. Take a little credit.

A: I'm a 'both and' gal.

E: But then there were still regressions. And there was something kind of under there. And it got to the point where I could almost see it, but I couldn't touch it, if that makes any sense. Whatever that thing was that I couldn't get to about myself, I don't know. I guess that's why the initial recommendation was made, right?

w: Well, it's got to a point with most of the people that I work with where it's very clear that they could continue with me, doing what I do, the way I push the agenda.

But at its core I know that, "Why should I put all this heavy lifting in and the person who I'm seeing has to put all this heavy lifting in for years sometimes?" And the sooner I can get him or her to a treatment that changes things, and ready them for that, the better. Because, sometimes, it can take years to ready a person; sometimes, it can be an initial encounter.

But I know that this is going to be the glue that is the catalyst for people to really get off the dime and make serious, big time changes. Because we know that this medicine work does that.

E: Oh, yeah.

W: And we know data-wise, even if we look at the data if you want to be scientifically driven, it's clear as a bell. We could wait for the phase three studies to start but...

A: But you said it wasn't what you expected.

E: No, not at all. Not even slightly. Not even slightly. So, you know obviously the setting, I feel very cool, like a cool guy doing it. It looks like Hemingway might live there. It's a very sort of cool enclave, and there's a lovely companion in the pup. And I had used MDMA before, well I had used methamphetamine masquerading as MDMA before. Nonetheless, it was quite a good time. So, I wasn't scared of the effects.

W: I even told him, I said to him, to everybody: Go in, at best, just have fun. You're allowed to have fun.

A: I may have said you have nothing to do.

E: You're right, you did say that. It's the truth. But the first forty-five minutes felt like three hours. Just nothing happened.

Obviously because it needs to kick in. And I believe that I mentioned to you at one point I had got a little cold, if I could have a blanket. And that nothing had happened. In my head, I'm like, no way this just goes bust and nothing happens today. That would suck.

And then we took the second dose. Finished some OJ. Laid down. And I figured, you know what, I'm tired. I'll take a nap. Maybe I'll take a nap, at the very least I'll get a good nap in today. So, I go into a sort of a curled-up ball like I normally sleep in, and not long after, or maybe very long after…I don't have a good sense of time in this whole thing. I have absolutely no sense to be honest.

You know it began as dark shapes, and colours started to move. Sort of when your eyes are dark, and you see those shapes. But they were more pronounced. The edges were harder, more defined than they had been. I remember feeling a bit of the electricity starting to kick in. I believe that would be the methamphetamine rushing through to keep you awake. And going on my back.

And the next thing I remember there's a creeping. There's a bit of light under the actual eye mask. I remember it just sort of growing and growing and growing and growing and getting impossibly bright. Not in a painfully overwhelming way. But in a very overwhelming way. And it got to the point where I was just fully encompassed in light, and there was absolutely nothing else anymore.

I believe at this point, somewhat far into this, I had been raising my arms up like this. And I do believe if I'm not mistaken, I asked you to help me stand up, so I could join that light.

A: Yes.

E: And upon sitting up, I realised, wow, sitting up quickly was a bad idea. And then standing was cool. The immediate thing I got for myself is it was very much a loud dialogue between me and me. And it was like a meeting with myself. It is a very apposite description. And it was like, you know, I understand that it's cool that you wanted to stand up and join this whole thing, and you needed that physical representation. But you also don't need it. If you're uncomfortable, you can just sit back down now. Yes, I would like to sit back down now. Thank you very much.

It was a very nonjudgmental but very honest analysis. I don't think that same analysis could have been done in a regular state of mind. I think the issues are too loaded with emotion and maybe pain.

So, the light continued to grow and continued to grow and continued to grow. One phrase I kept hearing was, "Don't you realise?" And then it would say this next thing, and I believe we spoke about this when I was here. It was rapid-fire, every single person in my entire life.

Like, "Don't you realise that you love your friend Sam because Sam is like this? He gives this to you and you give this to him and it's a great balance. And you both improve each other so much. Isn't it wonderful that you have this friendship?" Obviously. You know. "Don't you realise that the issue with your parents is this underlying thing. "

And it just blazes through this quickly. Like really with that amount of speed. But also precision. Like every single thing was like, Yep, Yep, Yep, Yep, Yep, Yep. Exactly right. All right, and then we're done. Just ripped through.

W: That takes care of years of therapy.

E: Exactly. And that was fun. But the real fun, the fun-fun started after that. I just kept going, and I just understood that we are a small blip on an everlasting beam of light. And this is just a small part of a journey which has taken a physical shape. And then I began to wonder why physical shapes exist, and why we would be in a way banished to a place where there would be suffering.

Then, I got to think of God, of course. And there's this old thing in Judaism that God had to retract some of himself because of pure everythingness. He had to pull back some of himself in order to allow the world to be created. I identified with that idea very strongly and noted that it was actually an amazing gift, because here we get the opportunity to sense something that really isn't, which is perfection. And meaningful perfection in a way that we can understand it is only a result of all the, frankly, imperfection, and if we're going to be more candid, the painful shit you face on such a routine basis. And that was overwhelming.

I also very strongly connected with a sage, one of the forefathers, Abraham. Avraham. The tale is he smashed these idols, because he recognised that idols were bullshit. And I came to see that as an analogy for my own lifelong obsession with money and success. And how I had commingled perfection-perfection with physical goods. And created this sort of death spiral where I assumed something poisonous was the ultimate goal of life. Right? And I understand why I got that mixed up. That's cool. It's not a big deal.

W: The odd thing is, perfectionist people tend to kill themselves more. I don't know if there's really truth to it, but there seems to be a semi-truth to it. It's more a statement metaphorically if you don't believe it.

E: It's an impossible bar to hold and hold.

W: And I gotta tell you something else. I don't think therapy in general or therapy in particular to you, would have ever revealed this. It couldn't have been revealed, and if it was revealed, it wouldn't have made any...

E: Made any sense. It wouldn't make sense. Like imagine if I was saying all this stuff to not you guys, but to people who had never done any of this before. You're nuts. Nuts. It's true, but it's nuts.

A: But that wonderful rapid-fire, "Don't you realise? Don't you realise?" Has that resulted in, can you feel any kind of ease from those, whatever they were?

E: Not only. It's more than an ease. And this is actually something I was going to call you about today anyway. But I have been so jacked up. Like every single day it's almost like the same thing happens again. It's brought me a tonne of calm and a lot of what I focused on was actually people in the workplace. Which you think you'd devote to old friends but no, it's a very honest experience. You devote it to whatever's actually on your head. You know, whatever is actually affecting you on a day-to-day basis, a lot of which is my job. So, I think about coworkers in absolute rapid-fire. But in the most...

W: How were thoughts about your coworkers, given this experience? How did it effect what we talked about in terms of keeping distance from them and playing a role with them? Not really showing yourself with them. All that discussion. Has that been impacted in some way?

E: It has. It has impacted. Because I'm separate, absolutely. Before we had talked about that. It was helpful, but it was cold. It came from an inherent place of negativity.

W: Yes.

E: I'm able to relate to people better, to act more like a professional. And at the same time, I've been able to show a lot more of my personality comfortably and in a way that I'm doing it from a place of positivity, not a place to show off. And it's better received. Obviously, everyone likes something more authentic, which when you're more comfortable, you're able to give over.

And I've realised a lot of my work, all of my work, is basically done with clients on the phone. I love talking on the phone. It's always enjoyable for me but I have just got much better at it. I diffused the most pissed off human being the other day. It was like a half an hour marathon with this guy going back and forth seven times with people today and he was having a rough day. And, I don't know. It increases your ability to have empathy toward difficult people while keeping in mind that not everyone is to be trusted.

A: You used the phrase jacked up a few moments ago.

E: Still jacked up. Yeah, it's got to the point where I'm like, is this supposed to stop? If it's going to stay like this, that would be the best. Does it stop?

A: It's absolutely an individual thing. The more open you become and the more you can accept that openness, the more you can maintain. There's no reason for it to stop because you're running on your own fuel now. It's not the medicine. This is you.

E: Is it out already?

A: Yes, it is.

W: Remember what Solomon said, you're doing the homework; you're maintaining the work. So, the thought process could continue and things could emerge in say six months, a year, because you read something. And it rejiggered up that stuff in your head that was there from this experience. And it starts all over again.

E: I noticed something the other day very strongly. I was at a couple of work outings one night. I had a decent bit to drink. Alcohol blocks the light, man.

W: I don't like drugs that close off too much. Though sometimes closing off is fine.

E: It can be. That's why, I don't know, I think the ability for people to like, drink wine at a wedding or something, I see that as such a beautiful thing now.

W: We know the rebbe's people would have these big gatherings where he would speak. And he would sing. Alcohol played a very prominent role. The rebbe himself would drink. Well, there are all sorts of discussions you and I could have about this.

That's why the work is ongoing and something that I think you and I, and you without me, you'll do it. Very much without me, you'll do it. And if you want to call, you'll call, you'll call me, you'll call Eli, but you'll do the work because it's an ongoing work and because you're philosophically inclined. Well, this will take you out of philosophy but it will certainly project you into spaces that you...

A: I think you said his philosophical training was a perfect foundation for this to happen.

E: Yes, it was. And I'd largely forgotten about all of it.

Actually, all of that stuff was good and well, but it wasn't visual. There was only one part that was truly like I was standing somewhere that I was not, physically. And that was definitely the pinnacle of the whole thing in terms of intensity. I had come out of this giant light and I was still beaming light, but I was in one of the halls at the Met (Metropolitan Museum, NYC). The one where there's all the Greek sculpture, and there's one where it's like a sculpture of a dude biting his hand because he knows he has to eat his children (Ugolino and His Sons). One very famous Greek sculpture there.

But I was in the hall. It's such a beautiful hallway; there's these amazing skylights. Light is absolutely pouring in. My realisation as I would shift, (and it was the same blazing efficiency) calculated everything. But this one was a little more measured because I was actually physically standing there looking around.

And what I realised is that beauty is not indicative of beauty. What does that mean? I'm still unpacking what that means. But something can be beautiful and still be wrong in this world. You can't measure things on this sliding scale of what is beautiful is good, what is ugly is bad. What is beautiful can be evil. What is ugly can be true. That barometer in and of itself is antithetical to the real perfection. The real perfection of things counting for their inner merit rather than their outer merit.

It doesn't matter how beautiful a marble statue is; if it's made with a bad intention, if it's made for the wrong reasons and all that, it's still a bad thing. You know, the energy is still bad. And at that point, and this I'm sad about still, I just had to go to the bathroom. Had to go to the bathroom. And I got back, I laid back down, I got the eyeshades on and I was like, dammit. It's gone. Can't go back to the Met.

So yeah, stupid bathroom. And I think I spoke to both of you about this that like, at a certain point your body is going to want to get you to do something else. You'll have an itch, you'll have a scratch, and you'll have to use the bathroom was the biggest one. I had to use the stupid bathroom. Dammit! I am actually pretty mad about that. As mad as you can be when you're happy about everything. Yeah!

w: I just can't resist. I've got to ask a question. How does that affect your life, the knowledge that beauty isn't always what it seems to be? In essence, may not be beautiful.

e: I'd love to unpack it, you know.

w: Okay.

e: I'd have to analyse it a little bit more. What I think it means is that a lot of the stuff I was fundamentally going for in life I was never fundamentally going for. That's probably why I wasn't getting to it.

W: What were you going for?

E: Money, stuff. I mean I got to reassess what is beautiful and what isn't, not based on what's shiny.

W: Did anybody notice anything about you this week or say anything to you about your behaviour or anything about you?

E: Let me see, a little bit, yeah. I've just been very energetic, you know? I can barely sit down. I love going to work out in a way that I very much used to. And I've had some actually very good feedback from people, especially with one girl from work who I ended up having a couple beers with and...Amazingly sweet person and in so much pain. From just abuse and illness and all this terrible shit that's befallen her. And honestly would have every excuse to be a complete mess, but is such a nice person, composed and professional.

And being able to really internalise what she was feeling even though we're from different backgrounds, different cultures, different everything, really. Different everything. Being able to just really connect with that in another person.

And the interesting thing is, to be quite honest, she's a beautiful girl. Really is. Physically, not just soul-wise, but there was no draw physically, which is odd. It was legitimately that I wanted to just know this person.

W: Okay.

E: And she noticed that as well.

W: Okay. Quickly, things I'm just going to go through. Have you talked to the ex-girlfriend at all?

E: No, but I want to. She's too blocked out by the world.

W: Do you have empathy for yourself?

E: Yeah. I need a little more of it. Sometimes I look in the mirror and I'll be like you should be really hitting the gym a little bit more. You really need a haircut, you really need this, you really need that. So, that stuff is still there. It's not like I'm all of a sudden the Zen-est person in the universe. I'm still a neurotic New York Jew. But I'm just a very happy neurotic New York Jew. And I cut myself more slack than I used to.

W: Do anything self-destructive this week?

E: I mean, I had a couple beers but I was bowling with some coworkers. That doesn't count. My level of self-destructive is I ate a bunch of grilled cheese with my friend when I was drinking.

W: Sounds good.

E: Oh, it was really good. It was brioche with olive bread. It was awesome.

W: Stop tempting me, it's Friday.

Walter's advocacy of this work is not unheard of but is hardly normative. His professional interest in and familiarity with prescription pharmacological solutions had led to his understanding of the healing potential of MDMA. He also has his own experience of working in non-ordinary consciousness, from which point of view he became able to suggest the medicine work, with adequate preparation, to select clients.

From a reading of their interaction here, the question arises: Could Elijah's experience with MDMA have been improved by outside interruptions from any individual? Clearly, the answer is no, it could not. The respectful silence he enjoyed throughout was the only condition that could have maintained his focus and enabled him to receive this breadth and depth of information from his psyche. Any interventions, however learned and well-meaning, whether verbal or tactile, would have brought him back to ordinary consciousness and resulted in a change in the trajectory of his session, as it had with his 'stupid bathroom' visit. His focus was enhanced in-session by his philosophical training that was in full operational mode, allowing him to examine what was happening within him even as it was happening. This skill also serves him well as he 'un-packs' the extraordinarily clarifying events he experienced.

CHAPTER FIVE

Unexperienced Experience

---

*"If you bring forth that which is within you,
that which you bring forth will save you.*

*If you do not bring forth that which is within you,
that which you do not bring forth will destroy you."*

THOMAS, THE GNOSTIC GOSPELS

Dr. Ivor Browne grew up in Ireland in the 1930s and 40s, and for him, the tension between the Protestant British and the Catholic Irish was not only political but personal: his mother was Protestant and his father, Catholic. During his medical training, he was bedridden with tuberculosis in both lungs for two, six-month periods; Ivor Browne's formative years were not easy.

As a young adult, Browne studied medicine at the College of Surgeons in Dublin. His career took him to several psychiatric hospitals, where he began to see how the traditional treatment system was failing its patients. Browne worked at the Grangegorman Mental Hospital and Saint John of God's Psychiatric Hospital in Dublin, the Warneford Hospital in Oxford and the Marlborough Day Hospital in London before winning a scholarship to study in the United States, accepting a position as a psychiatric intern at Massachusetts General Hospital in 1960. During his time in the United States, Browne was exposed to psychoactive compounds that introduced him to non-ordinary consciousness and opened him to the vastness of the human psyche. He carried that understanding with him when he returned to Ireland in 1962 to take up a position of chief psychiatrist to the Dublin Health Authority.

While working with traumatised patients, he hypothesised that when the psyche perceives the traumatic violation as an extreme, potentially mortal threat to the organism itself, it: 1) creates a non-ordinary state of consciousness; and 2) captures the memory of the trauma to prevent further threat to the victim. This extraordinary event prevents the victim from having any coherent access to the event or events, which remains, in Browne's words, 'incohate' within the body. Under life-threatening duress, the psyche reacted instantaneously by capturing the threat and cordoning it off, where it cannot be remembered. There it stays suspended, denied, and unexperienced.

Significantly, the traumatic memory is caught and held at an extremely high threat level, a level sufficient for the psyche to understand that the organism could be damaged by having to experience the trauma, precipitating its original action to capture the memory. It faithfully carries this protection going forward, but because it remains at the dreadful peak of the traumatic experience, it does so with great difficulty. The tight hold the psyche must maintain forestalls any possibility that the fear of the event can ever be fully experienced. In this condition, it can never be fully understood by the organism in a way that would allow for a diminution of the threat level, potentially leading to release and completion. The traumatic event remains at its peak threat-level intensity, caught and held within the body by the psyche's capture, but may be entirely unknown to us. The experience is cut off from us, and as Dr. R. D. Laing has expressed, we become cut off from the fact that it has been cut off. Yet, we know about it somatically from our symptoms, even if we don't cognitively know that we know.

An example of this action might be a rape victim who has amnesia about the event itself and is unable to describe the attacker, his clothes, or any other details that might be reasonably expected under normal circumstances. They are mute, because this is anything but normal circumstances. The content is no longer available to them, because when their emotional fear escalated to the maximum life-threatening level during the rape, greater than anything the victim may have experienced before, the organism understood this as a mortal threat and immediately and decisively cut off all normal access to memory of the event. The person endured and survived the trauma, yet, even though the psyche had banished the event from their conscious memory, the effects of the attack are still imprinted in the body. The threat is not available for recall either by short-term or long-term memory, yet it exists inchoate within the body.

We go forward from such a traumatic event doing the best we can to operate with the threat still held within us, until we are triggered in a situation that frightens us. We may be hypersensitive to relatively harmless events that our bodies translate into lethal threats akin to the original trauma. We may have radically inappropriate responses to minor disturbances, restless nights immersed in nightmares or reacting with terror during Guy Fawkes Day or Fourth of July fireworks. Post-traumatic stress symptoms may occur, because trigger-events send us right back into the original traumatic moment. We're no longer celebrating; we are back in Iraq facing an (IED) explosion.

What is happening here? Essentially, the body, which still carries the captured memories of the event, even as they are hidden from us, no longer wants this burdensome chore and uses every opportunity to shed the load. Trigger responses may occur at any moment, precluding any possibility of our being able to process them, and we experience them as annoying symptoms, or worse. Yet, symptoms are signals, messages from the body alerting us to an underlying condition requiring our attention. These very symptoms are, in fact, artefacts of the body's ongoing project to make every attempt to bring this condition to our attention and to relieve itself of the terrible secrets it holds.

The repercussions of trauma run deep, and it is well beyond our conscious ability to understand quite how deep. If you are traumatised very young, you carry the wound in your growing body where not only is every new cell affected by contact, the brain circuitry has also been affected by the trauma. It is in this condition that the victim of trauma is effectively condemned to live, believing, in the absence of any real information, that the problem is endogenous *to* them. It is not; the problem is exogenous and only lies *within* them. We do not live in the past; the past lives in us. The horror has been internalised very effectively, concealed more deeply than we can comprehend and from this point of view, we feel it is actually us.

It is not.

All the while, the body desperately wants to get rid of this secret but cannot find an effective way to do so. To the body, the crisis is constantly present, an as-yet unexperienced experience.

Dr. Ivor Browne's description of traumatic memory as the frozen present rings true. We carry it, frozen, throughout our lives until we act to give it the opportunity to be released. To heal, our primary task is to put ourselves in a situation where we trust that we are without a doubt safe, and this is precisely what we do when we offer ourselves to this medicine work.

The psyche doesn't comprehend time. Like everything else within our skin-encapsulated body, it lives hypervigilant in the eternal Now, from which timeless position it responded instantaneously to the original threat, capturing the memory in order to protect us. Lacking further instructions from any quarter, it faithfully maintains its hold on the memories going forward, attempting to release them by opportunistically seizing on environmental and other triggers to do so. When acting from our own agency we give the psyche its best opportunity to reveal the traumatic memory for our consideration; it then releases itself from the responsibility it has carried since saving our lives. We, ourselves, move into the present moment, where there is no threat. The organism can now understand this for the first time, unclench its fist, and release the trauma, restoring our psychic balance.

That's exactly the opportunity clients have in the treatment room; to be able to move into the present moment so the trauma can be released. We provide an environment that is completely relaxed; the room, itself, and every element immediately outside the client's body is free and clear of anything but the attendant's full attention, love, and support. As far as possible, a timeless atmosphere that accords with the timeless body is created and maintained, an environment free of any exogenous influences; no advice, suggestions, prompts, input from disciplines like philosophy or religion, psychology or psychiatry, or helpful tips need intrude. The atmosphere outside the client's immediate external space is clear and pure, giving the maximum possible internal time and psychic space for the client to engage with information emerging from within them, allowing engagement, ownership, and release.

The client rests in a completely safe setting with someone they trust, and in this condition, the psyche is presented with a unique opportunity to understand that the organism is no longer under threat. During these moments of the session, the psyche's attention is withdrawn from its mono-focus on maintaining its hold on the captured memories to include the reality it is now experiencing—that the organism is safe and well. Once this is established, the psyche acts according to the same principle of protection that caused it to capture the traumatic memory in the first instance; finding there is no longer anything to protect, it reverses itself and releases the traumatic memory. This may be partial, requiring further sessions, or complete, as the interested reader will see within some of the testimonies.

Because it understood we were at risk, the psyche originally acted to protect the organism by capturing the memory of the traumatic wound and shutting it out of our memory. By deliberately preparing an environment where in every moment there is no present threat, the psyche can reconsider its role. The mono-focus it has dutifully maintained is supplanted by a dual-focus, or bifurcation, wherein the psyche can see the event from both points of view; it *was* horrific, but this *is* not. In its ever-present modus operandi of Now, it understands that it is not 1992 anymore, and that the client is now safely established on a couch supported with love and attention. Within the non-ordinary consciousness created by the medicine, the psyche is then able to realise this changed circumstance now present within the organism and can open the closed fist with which it has been holding onto the memory of the trauma, and release it.

For the client, this may be the first time they remember the trauma itself without being entirely overwhelmed. The content is now available to them, as well as the associated feelings, but the fear no longer engulfs them. The memory may raise some anxiety going in, but it is manageable as the client knows he or she is safe and also has somebody to support them. In-session, they live simultaneously in both realities—the reality of the present and the reality of the past.

The effect of releasing trauma is evident in clients' daily lives following treatment. They can go forward able to describe and understand the event as a normal, recallable memory, and can integrate this understanding into their lives. One client tells how she has forgiven everyone involved in the violence done to her as a child and is now able to get on with her life. She can use the information she uncovered; she can talk about her dysfunctional teenage and young adult years with clarity and without sinking back into shame and depression. Now, the memories brought to the surface can serve as information-rich tools for further healing, rather than weapons that reinforce the original scar.

Such cognitive processing, however, remains secondary to the action of the medicine on the body. The somatic release is the main event, and everything we do as attendants is to enable the release by maintaining a neutral environment.

Dr. Peter Levine has worked with trauma all his life and describes how wild animals recover from trauma. He cites a cheetah on the savannah in Africa, chasing an impala. As the cheetah leaps, the impala may fall before it's even captured, behaving as if it is already dead. In this moment, the impala has entered a non-ordinary state of consciousness in which it just accepts whatever is going to happen. This course of action may also save its life, because the cheetah, who is uninterested in dead prey, often walks away. Then, the impala may rise, alive and unharmed. It shakes its body convulsively, as if to throw off the whole experience and returns to the herd.

What Levine describes in animals is an example of the biological release mechanism available to all sentient beings. We humans, with all our cleverness and thinking, have completely overlooked and ignored the value of entering a non-ordinary state of consciousness that may lead to the automatic response, shaking out the trauma that comes naturally to other creatures. One way we do accomplish a similar release is through movement—sport, dance, and exercise. Eastern exercise forms such as Chi Gong, interestingly, include shaking exercises. Levine's somatic experiencing explores this healing mechanism with shaking and various techniques to ameliorate and release trauma. Some people have success with other somatic methods like EMDR that can also present us with hidden traumatic memories for processing and recalibration.

Dr. Ivor Browne understood the physical release phenomenon from his own experiences in non-ordinary consciousness, and he observed it in some of his patients who had been exposed to psychoactive medicines prior to their prohibition. Browne worked with some of the most difficult cases, people who had been given up by the psycho-medical system as hopeless, and in this way brought them back to emotional and physical balance.

He observed the reactions of seriously mentally ill people in non-ordinary consciousness and observed their positive outcomes following release of their traumatic memories. They were finally experiencing the unexperienced. His understanding that we can only accomplish this release in a non-ordinary state of consciousness that parallels the non-ordinary state consciousness experienced during capture of the original trauma is the key and essential insight of his elegant hypothesis, Psychological Trauma, or Unexperienced Experience. It is a truism that to know ourselves, we must step outside our everyday way of processing the world. As Albert Einstein observed, "We cannot solve our problems with the same thinking we used when we created them."

To our witness, the transformations that occur in MDMA sessions affirm Browne's hypothesis unequivocally, and the mechanism-of-action of his hypothesis is also acknowledged by researchers in the field.

Morton Herskowitz, author of *Emotional Armouring*, says, "It is axiomatic in medicine that theories proliferate when the disease is not comprehended. Once the cause is known and the process is understood, the multiplicity ceases." It is our sincere hope that this book, through the testimonies of individuals, may help to demonstrate the validity of Browne's hypothesis of unexperienced experience. To our view, the embrace of this neglected hypothesis is essential if we are to understand the actual mechanisms that underlie trauma capture and release, and to clarify our currently problematic relationship with trauma.

If we misunderstand the cause of the problem, we are bound to fail with our chosen treatment. Take, as an example, one common PTSD symptom—getting into fights. In seeking to extinguish the behaviour, conventional treatment addresses the end result, the behaviour itself, with pharmacology (drugs), cognitive behavioural therapy, etc. This symptom-centric approach may be necessary to protect the public peace, but critically absent is any real understanding of the underlying cause or examination of its source. The individuals themselves may not know why they have overwhelming impulses to punch people's lights out. They think this is just who they are.

When criticisms and punishments pile up in an effort to curb the negative behaviours, people, understandably, take it personally. If this is who they are, and who they are is deemed unacceptable, then they have yet another reason to be angry and resistant. In these instances, experiencing the vicious cycle they are in, they may come to believe there is no possibility of help from any quarter.

It does not need to be so painful and lonely, but we need to show up for ourselves. After the unexperienced experience is brought forth and released, the troubling symptomatic behaviours may resolve themselves. People who have experienced this release tell in their testimonies how their problem behaviour was reduced or stopped entirely. Once the *cause* of their sympto-mological behaviour has been reduced or eliminated, they just do not feel compelled to do the fighting, drinking, or drug-ging anymore.

Modern medicine focuses almost entirely on eliminating symp-toms, which are the body's way of alerting us to an underlying problem. We kill the messenger. Little encouragement is given to look for the root cause of a problem. If you have a headache, you will likely be told to take some aspirin. You take the pill, the headache goes away, and you feel better. Except that you will get another headache again soon, because nobody has asked why you get headaches. Maybe they are precipitated by tension from a difficult work environment or too many video games. If you changed jobs or reduced your playtime, would your headaches go away forever? You might not even consider it, because the pharmaceutical 'remedy' is always close at hand.

Not only can experiencing the root cause of the problem result in its release and cause the symptoms to disappear, it also helps prevent people from falling victim to future trauma. The terrible irony is that traumatised people are often unconsciously drawn to situations that provoke their symptoms, keeping the cycle of trauma rolling on and on, even inter-generationally. If, on the other hand, we can correct and even eliminate the primal cause, the need for this repetitive behaviour to occur may be eliminated.

When we are done with the trauma, the trauma is done with us.

I used to have bad dreams a lot, like explosions in my sleep.

Sgt. K.

To sit with a war veteran as they revisit the traumatic events of their service is an extraordinary lesson; what these young men and women have endured is beyond endurance. To bear witness to the unfolding of their personal horror, experienced as it was in the war zone within the ever-present fear of their own imminent mortality, is to appreciate in some small measure what it is to serve in the line of fire and to be humbled by one's own lack of courage to do so.

Sgt. K. served both before and after 9/11, until the ambush that ended his military career. He survived with a wicked back and a diagnosis of PTSD, finding his way through the thicket of conflicting advice from the Veterans Administration (VA) and eventually to this work. I am personally grateful to have been able to be present for him and to witness the return to his familiar and deserving self; a loving son, father, and husband.

Why and when did you decide to join the Marines?

It was in 1996, when I was twenty-one or twenty-two. I was making six dollars an hour doing plumbing, and I hated it. I just wanted to leave for a while and do something hard, so I tried that. All the knuckleheads in my family go into the military.

So, first you went for training?

I was in Camp Lejeune (Marine Corps Base Camp in Jacksonville, North Carolina) for the first year of boot camp, and then I went to infantry school. It was cool; I had a lot of good friends. There's a lot of good guys in the military. It's not like the regular world—the civilian world. You have people to count on.

You felt that people really had your back?

Yeah, and they know everything about you.

Is that because you're in such close quarters?

I guess it's because it sucks so much, and you're going through it together. Combat is like a high. You never feel more alive knowing you could die at any second. And I notice that there are two different kinds of people—the ones who go once and never ever want to go again. And the ones who want to keep going all the time.

And which category do you fall into?

The second one, unfortunately. I got out in 2000, but then 9/11 happened, and I signed back up.

What made you leave the military in 2000?

There was nothing going on. I was tired of getting yelled at all the time. I was done; I did my time. But once 9/11 happened, it was like, once a Marine always a Marine. They got you brainwashed good. Also, I knew my unit was getting activated. We were supposed to go to Afghanistan, but we went to Camp Lejeune for a year to train, then we went home for a month or two, and then I got called up for Iraq. So, I went to Iraq in 2003, and then in 2004, I was out. But I wasn't really functioning too good in the regular world. All I could think about was going back. Fallujah was going on that year. I got obsessed; it was my life.

So, you returned to the states in 2004 but then decided to go back to Iraq?

I was looking for a unit to deploy with. I found a unit that was in West Virginia, so I joined that one in 2005. But it was bad that time; the second time in Iraq was much worse.

So, you were in Iraq twice?

Yeah.

Can you tell me what the first time was like?

People would take potshots at you, but they weren't very accurate. You were worried going in, because they would shoot scuds at us from Kuwait, and you gotta run to a sandpit, put your mask on and hope it doesn't land on you. But I would've much rather slept in bed and just died in my sleep than run out every time a scud went off. It was annoying. You'd be in chemical suits too. Remember in `03 we thought we were gonna be getting gassed. But that whole thing we made up.

— I hope I never see blood like
  that again.
— Blood everywhere. Kid's
  shot, Marines.
— I'll show you. I'll be a grunt.
  You didn't go to Vietnam.
  I'll go to Iraq twice.
— If Joey was here, what would
  he say? He'd tell me to get
  right back at it.
— Just beautiful. I'm so lucky.
— There's a Vet with a gun
  in his mouth somewhere,
  looking at his bottle of pills.
— Some people can hold this
  in for 10 years.

Notes taken by the attendant during Sgt. K's first session.

That was all made up?

Well, we never found any chemical weapons.

Did you ever worry for your safety?

Not me, because I always thought it's not gonna happen to me. Until it happens to you, and then you think about it a lot. It's pretty real. It's Darwinian I guess; you live or you die, that's it.

What happened? Did you have any very bad incidents?

Yeah, a whole bunch. I got blown up in a vehicle and my friend, Joey, he died. So, that was a shit show. It was crazy. It was something else, really. We had just turned a corner and were going down this road and we hit a mine. Two of the guys flew into the air. I was looking at them like, what happened? They got ejected. My friend was in bad shape. He was bleeding internally, and he was all crooked and with stuff on his face; he looked the wrong way. I knew it wasn't good. We tried to get helicopters, but they couldn't land, because there was a humongous sandstorm, and it had started to rain. It took over two hours to get him to the hospital. They were trying to get him to a base where he could get operated on. But he died in the air, in the helicopter.

Did you get injured as well?

Yeah, five of us were in the hospital. The driver got a bad concussion. I was treating my friend, Jake, after we got blown up, because the doc was working on my friend, Trembley, as he was really bad. It blew up right underneath him. I thought my friend, Jake, was dead, but he wasn't; he was in shock. I was holding his tongue while I was talking to my friend Joey. They landed right next to each other. I got a little shrapnel in my leg; it was nothing. We were all in the hospital. And the last time I saw Joey, he was flopping around on a table with a sheet over his waist, and I was talking to him. I was yelling, telling them to help him and shit. I was pretty high on morphine too. I remember they said he was gonna be all right. And then the chaplain woke me up and told us that he died. If we could've landed the helicopter, if there was no sandstorm, he might've lived.

So, you're in the hospital, and you're being treated for your wounds. What happened to you?

I had hairline fractures in my vertebrae. I had a pinched nerve. I went to the VA after, and they said I'm always gonna have a bad back. But I made it through. It sucked. My guys would look out for me though; they'd try to carry extra stuff of mine. I was stubborn though too, trying to lead by example. But yeah, all my Marines were awesome. I love those guys. It's the people, the guys—that's what it is.

Why did you return to the US after your second time in Iraq?

My son. He gave me a new mission. Physically you burn out quick in the Marines. It's like football—physical. And then I had my son, so there was no reason to go anymore really. I was old when I got blown up. I hurt my back; I was in the hospital for like eleven days. They kept me so high for those days. And I had five more months to do, and I didn't want to go home. I wanted to help my Marines. I didn't want any of my other Marines to die. They were all young; I was old. So, I was worried about them. Because when I went there the first time, my sergeant always looked out for me, and now that was my job. I had to finish my job, otherwise I would've had to go back a third time. But I was in a lot of pain and it took everything to make it through the five months. Wearing all that gear—sixty pounds of gear with a bad back. I couldn't physically do the job anymore. It's a young man's thing—that's why they always send them, unfortunately.

So, when you returned to the US, what was it like for you being back?

The second time I tried to make it work, because I didn't want to end up how I was the first time when I came home. I basically lived in an apartment with a bed on the floor and a TV on a milk crate, and I drank a lot. And all I thought about was going back.

Were you working at all when you got back?

Yeah, I've always been working. It's weird to go from combat patrol to working at Coca-Cola. It seems meaningless sometimes. You go over to Iraq, drop million-dollar bombs and stuff. I guess I still get to kill people though because I work for Coca-Cola [laughs].

Indirectly! [laughs]

Slowly.

When you got back the first time, did you do any sort of therapy or support work within the VA?

No. Beer.

Beer was your therapy?

Yeah. And then I went to the VA the second time, because I was like, 'Oh I'll just suck it up the last five months of my deployment and when I get home, the VA will take care of me.' But, oh, no. They don't take care of you. I know guys that have gone to the VA and died in VA care.

Really. From what?

Pills. So, I don't want to have anything to do with the VA.

Can you tell me more about your experience with the VA.

Ugghh...it makes me so mad. They were always trying to give me pills, even though they didn't know anything about me. They just see me and think, "Oh, this guy has a purple heart, and he got blown up, so let's give him something." Like crazy pills. But I always said no. I never wanted pills. I'm not the smartest guy in the world, but that was probably the smartest decision I've ever made. Thank God for that, really. Because guys I know that do the pills, they're in bad shape. They give them like ten different ones, too. Some make you happy, some make you want to kill yourself, some are for your high blood pressure. And a lot of these guys have physical pain and ailments too, and they're getting like Oxy's and stuff. So, now you're hooked on those things, and from what I've seen, it's bad. Because it doesn't work.

And those are the people shooting people, too. They don't read the side effects; they just take it. And the guys who drink, they're bad too. After the first time I came home, my sergeant killed himself. Nobody saw that one coming. I don't want any of my other friends committing suicide, drinking their faces off. I have one friend who is always drunk. It's terrible. But the weed guys are good. I'm in that one. But for real, that helped me a lot. For the ten years until I met the attendant, weed would help me relax. It was good. There was one nice lady at the VA. and she offered to help me, to talk to me, because she was nice. Even she told me that weed could help but that she wasn't allowed to say that. Weed was helping me survive. Definitely. After everybody went to sleep, I could smoke a bowl, and I would actually have some calm and quiet. It would help me fall asleep too.

So, you went to the VA, and all they could offer you was pills?

They give you pills and a heating pad, because I couldn't do physical therapy because of work. It sucks. I hate it. It makes me mad, really. It feels like they used us for our bodies and our minds, and now they're trying to profit off these guys for what, their whole life with pills, ten pills a day? It's like a big pharmacy, right? It makes me mad when they could just do MDMA. You only have to do it a couple times and you're good.

What was going on with you physically and mentally when you returned home after your last time in Iraq?

You have to process everything that you just went through, because when you're in Iraq, shit happens, and you gotta go and do it. Like, recently, they burned a guy to death in a cage, right? I recovered like sixteen burning bodies once. They were contractors, and they got ambushed bad. Like, IEDs, mortars, RPGs, AK-47s, everything. Everything. So, we had to go get their bodies, and when we got there, they were skeletons on fire. I'll never forget the smell in the back of the vehicle. It smelled like 9/11. And you'd see the bodies in the cars, melting. So, we had to get the burned bodies and put them in body bags. And the

Iraqis working with the contractors were also executed. They stacked their bodies up and booby-trapped them with a bomb, so whoever would take the bodies off would get hit with a bomb. But my friend saw the booby trap, and then we had to shoot a hellfire missile at the bodies to blow up the IED. So, little things that happen every day can take you back.

Also, nightmares. I used to have bad dreams a lot, like explosions in my sleep. It still happens sometimes. I had one the other night, where my house was being overrun by ISIS (the Islamic State of Iraq and Syria) guys. And me and my sister fought them all off. And my sister, who would never touch a gun in her whole life, was like Rambo. I would have bad dreams a lot. My wife will never wake me up if I'd fall asleep on the couch, because I don't like to be startled. And I still don't like crowds.

How was your wife able to handle all that you were going through?

The first time I came back, she left for a while. The second time, I was pretty good. It's been a process, you know. I could be abrupt. I get quiet. I'm like a clam too—the longer I stay quiet, I'll just stay quiet. It's never been one of my strong suits, I guess. And I'm stubborn.

Were you able to share what you were going through with her?

I have in the past, but now I don't. Because I feel like she doesn't understand really. I think she feels I should just forget about it. It's the worst thing, really. But she's gotta take care of my son and shit, too. It's crazy. She's awesome though. She's a good person. I'm just saying, it's not something you can forget really. I wish I could. But it made me who I am now—well, that's how I look at it. It made me who I am, and I survived. I'm a scrawny white guy, but I'm pretty tough. Not that my friends weren't. We lost forty-eight Marines. My unit lost the most Marines out of anybody who's been to Iraq or Afghanistan. It's not something you really want to be known for. There was a lot of death.

What led you to MDMA?

Ha! Ten years. I did everything, too. I did the VA; I did weed; I'd go for walks. I did acupuncture. I got to the point where I was functioning, but I was in turmoil all day long, and it was exhausting. I was so tired. I just wanted to be better. So, this is how it went down. My mom is a nurse, and she knows this doctor who's a family friend. He wrote me a prescription for Marinol, which is THC, for off-label purposes, because you can't get it for PTSD, which is crazy. It should be criminal. So, he checked me out and suggested I talk to this psychologist. Somehow, this psychologist was into MDMA, and he would send me stuff once in a while about it. But I was in denial still. I was like, "I'm all right, I got this." That's a big problem with military guys; we have the suck-it-up mentality. And 'don't be a sissy' kinda thing. But then, it seemed like a cycle kept happening. Sometimes, I can tell when it's happening, but if I can't, it will last a long time, maybe weeks.

What do you mean by cycle?

Where you just feel horrible. My brain would be working, like grinding gears constantly. It'd be exhausting trying to work and raise my son and do everything else. I was doing it, but it was getting hard. It was really hard. It's so hard to put into words what it was like. It was like a nagging brain injury. So, when the

psychologist brought up MDMA to me again, I said, "I'll do it."
And that's when I met my attendant.

So, this psychologist took you to meet an MDMA therapist?

Yeah. So, I met him, and a month later took MDMA, and it was
fucking awesome. I felt something leave my body, like a weight.
I'm not like perfect or anything, but I felt like I let the weight go
from my hands. Seriously. I knew I was reaching up, and I asked,
"Was I reaching up?" It felt like a huge burden was lifted. And I
could feel love for the first time in a *long* time. I always knew my
mom loves me, and my wife loves me, and my son loves me. I
know it, but on MDMA, I felt it. It was crazy; it was sick. And it
just made me think about a lot of stuff from Iraq. I don't know
what it did, man. War is hate and anger and confusion and tense.
It's constant, and it's relentless. But MDMA has got the love; it's
the only thing that can knock it out.

What a nice way to put it.

My head is so much clearer now. I can function during the day.
That's one of the biggest things that I notice; I'm much more
clear-headed, and I can live in the moment more. When I think
about the past, I still think about what happened. But I won't
stay on it forever, "perseverate" is the word they used to tell me
at the VA. I can just let it go, or I can think about my friends in
positive ways, or the fun ways or the funny ways. It helped. And
I always thought I was gonna die. All the time I'm out here, I feel
like I'm gonna die; someone's gonna kill me.

Even back home you were paranoid and worried about your
safety?

Yeah, I never felt safe. I would think something's gonna happen and who's gonna take care of my son if I'm killed out here? Or what if I get sick and die? I don't know why.

So, you were always living with fear of death?

Yeah, and then I did MDMA. And my attendant was like, "That's because that's how you lived in Iraq every day." And I was like, why couldn't I see that myself? But now, I'm not thinking I'm gonna die, really. It was a huge burden. It's weird. The next day, I was fine.

Did you have any fear going into your first MDMA session?

I was afraid at first. I was nervous. I had to lay on a couch, and I had this pink eye mask on, and I'm like, "Jesus Christ, this guy's gonna harvest my organs." [laughs] So, first, I started feeling it in my hands and in my feet, and then you just start feeling great. My hands are usually sore, because I use my hands every day. And they felt awesome, and my feet and my back felt awesome. Everything I touched was like, "Wow, this wall feels awesome." Water tasted awesome. I just felt so happy. Seriously, I never felt happy and relieved like that. I don't know what it was doing. It feels like you're not supposed to be that happy, regularly. Well, you don't let yourself be that happy. I could feel my mother, my son, and my wife. I could feel how much they loved me. There was a colour of black and red, too. It was awesome.

What's the significance of the black and red?

I don't know. It was like a pattern. It was kind of like a flooding. I know you don't really hallucinate. I don't know what was going on, but it was awesome. I felt their love; I could see it; I could feel it with all of my senses. Wow, it's cool, because when you're in combat, all your senses are the same too. I can smell it; I can see it. You use a lot of your senses, but in a good way with the MDMA. I probably went over that accident in Iraq. I just went off and my attendant listened. I had never really spoken to anybody about it really. And he's a really good listener. I got on a roll about a lot of stuff. About my friend. I don't know how many incidents I talked about with him. There are so many. After I did it the first time, I was like, "I feel like there's something else." I felt like I had to go again. And when I did, it made me realise that I didn't have to be afraid for my life all the time. That was the second time I went. And that was really good.

Were you just revisiting your time in Iraq or did you go into your childhood at all?

No, it was mostly about Iraq. My first session, I talked about my friend Joey a lot, a lot. I miss him. We became friends right away. We were the only two guys from my county in the West Virginia unit. He was an awesome Marine. He's somebody you'd want to watch your back.

Did you have any anxiety during the session?

No, I loved it. I didn't have any bad feelings the whole time. I was so thirsty though. I must've drank over a gallon of water. I was so thirsty. I drank so much water; I was peeing and everything.

Did you have any side effects the next day? Headaches?

I had a little bit of a sore throat, both times. But it went away the next day. I think, maybe, because I was so thirsty. I wasn't whacked out. I was good.

So, would you consider your experience 100 percent positive? There was nothing bad about it?

There was no bad part. I can't think of anything.

And even when you were revisiting these really horrific scenes from your time in Iraq?

Yeah, I was all right. Once it kicked in, it was almost like I knew how to use it in a way. It just did its work. I didn't really have to do much. I got a little choked up a few times.

Do you feel like you're more in touch with your emotions as a result of the work?

Yeah. I felt like I didn't have feelings for ten years a lot of the time. I can appreciate little things like, anything, just waking up, going to work. Even if it sucks, at least I'm out working. Even when it's over, you can get stuff from it. Does that make sense?

Completely.

I had a lot of stress lately. It was a little rough, but it's no big deal. I got through it. Now, only little things nag—you know, regular life. But yeah, it was a really positive experience. Nothing bad at all.

After your first session, why did you feel that you wanted to do it again?

I felt like I wasn't done. I felt like there was more. I felt like I could do it even better the next time, because I don't have to worry if my attendant is gonna do something to me! (laughs). I knew what was gonna happen. The first time, I didn't know what was gonna happen. The feeling in my hands and in my feet, I didn't know that was gonna happen. The second time, I was like, all right, here it is, it's coming. Do your thing. I'm just going to lay here.

And what emerged during your second session?

Well, the big thing that helped me was I realised that I was living like I was in Iraq still. I don't have to be afraid for my life all the time. And I'm not the same. Everybody used to be like, "Oh, you're not the same, you're not the same." Like, no I'm not. No shit! No shit! I'm not. Leave me alone. I'm all right though, I'm good. You go there! Plus, everybody changes over time, right? I've been home for ten years. Everything changes. But I always felt I had to be who I was before. It's not happening. Plus, I'm much smarter now, for crying out loud. That's for sure. I used to feel bad about my service, but MDMA made me realise who I am. I'm tough, and I can survive. I can keep going. My friend wouldn't want me to be a mess. He doesn't want that. He has probably been watching me as it is. And I want to be a good dad, make my son proud, and my friend proud, and be a better husband. And I want to enjoy my life. I'm forty. I'm almost dead. It goes like that (snaps his fingers). I got grey hairs. It doesn't last forever. You're not promised tomorrow. So, it's changed me for sure. It's so good, I don't understand what the problem with MDMA is.

Given your experience with the VA, do you think they'll ever be open to this?

No, the VA is so fucked up. The system would have to break, I feel. When you go to the VA, it's cold, it's dingy. You go to work with MDMA, it's *Night at the Museum*. A friggin' awesome dog who knows when you're peaking on your MDMA. What a difference between the two places! You go in the VA hospital, and it's so scary, man. You see the old guys in there. And I feel like they want us like that too. They want us zombied out, strung out. Because they know we know they're full of shit and they know we know how to use guns.

Do you feel that's what happens when you go to war—that most of the returning Marines understood that maybe they weren't being told the truth about the war?

A lot of us knew when we were there, but we didn't give a shit after a while. We know that nobody at home cares about this; they're bored with this. And we're just here to get through our time, and we're gonna make it. And that's all you care about. It doesn't matter what people think. People say they support the troops. I don't want a magnet on the back of your car with a yellow ribbon. Give `em MDMA! I don't want your car magnet. Donate your three dollars to MAPS (The Multidisciplinary Association for Psychedelic Studies) or something.

Now I feel like a lot of people are afraid of veterans. I don't like that. I was in class the other day, and they were talking about who is a minority group that's discriminated against. And they were all guessing. And my teacher's like, "No, no, no, no. It's veterans." They won't get hired because they're like, "Oh, when's this guy gonna snap?" And they were asking the kids in the class their point of view on veterans. They said, "They're violent" or "They're crazy." I was just sitting there like, "Wow, this is what people are starting to think of us."

And I don't want guys to suffer, it's not right. These guys gave their bodies and their minds. Their hearts were in the right places, even if the government wasn't doing the right thing. These guys were all kids that joined after 9/11, like the WWII guys. It's the same thing. It's just less of us now. They just want to send the same guys over and over and think that everything's going to be okay. It's not gonna be okay. It's not even fair to do multiple deployments. It should be a once-in-a-lifetime thing. That's why I tell my son, "I went once for me, and I went once for you. We're good."

And do you feel you want to do MDMA again?

Yeah, I feel like I should do it once a year.

Have you told anybody about your MDMA experience?

We had a reunion a couple of years ago. If we had another one, I definitely would tell more friends. Plus, they know I'm kinda...I'm not a hippie, but I'm more open-minded in some ways.

I wondered if you told people that they would call you a hippie [laughs]. Because that's just what you get called automatically when you talk too much about emotions and love.

Oh, yeah! Even when I said it before, I thought to myself, "Oh, please, Mr. Hallmark." But I know a couple guys too who really could use some MDMA. [Leans close into the microphone] "EVERYBODY SHOULD DO MDMA."

We'll put that in caps [laughs]. It's an amazing position to be in, going through this work and how well you've come out of it.

I know, but I don't understand why nobody knows about it. It's really sad.

Really sad. I think that so many of us who have done this work feel that Ugghhh, if only we had access to this years ago, we could've been younger and....

The VA should be giving it out. It's like, "Come to the VA for two days, and we'll have a party for you, and you'll be all right." Take MDMA [snaps his fingers] and boom! Six hours, changes your life. Guys would go! There's proof too. I'm sure you've read all of it since you've done it.

I've read every article.

MAPS and Reset.me. I just think veterans, anybody. Man, even if nothing's wrong with you, I think you should try it once. People will take anything else. They'll take Prozac or anything if it has a 'Z' in it, it's okay. All right then, so we'll call it Exta-Z [laughs].

The frustration Sgt. K. expresses with the unavailability of this medicine to help his brothers and sisters in-arms is righteous. As he says, he found his way to this work 'by luck' and for him to see his fellow service members suffering and suicidal for lack of access to this method of release from PTSD is to pour salt on already terrible wounds. He is committed to working for MDMA to be removed from the Schedule I designation it currently has, and just as he did while in service, to do his loyal best to honour and protect his buddies.

His e-mail sign-off is the measure of the man: 'Peace and good things.'

• • •

What was behind all the feelings I was having?

J.

J. was referred by a professional familiar with trauma, and when I met him at the intake consultation, he spoke so rapidly and in such expansive and exotic circumlocutions, it was very hard to make coherent sense of his narrative. He spoke of following rock bands, of 'eating' LSD, of crushing his foot in a motorcycle accident and other misadventures from a thoroughly marginal life. His first session was a physical, emotional, and psychic revisit to the sexual abuse that had reversed the trajectory of his youth from one of academic and athletic promise to one of torpor, indifference, and lack of ambition. His father despaired at this unaccountable change in his beloved son. J. completed high school, but in spite of obvious talent, he never attended college, able only to embark upon an outsider, off-the-grid life.

When I came to the work, I had been sober from alcohol and hard drugs for just over three years, about three years and four months. Prior to that, I had substance abuse problems. A recurring issue in my life was that from age fourteen or fifteen through thirty-two, although I got sober at age twenty and was sober for the majority of my adult life, I had a number of different periods of really intense substance abuse and poly-substance abuse. I was doing a lot of different drugs at the same time. After a series of events in my early thirties, I started to have really strong PTSD symptoms, which led to my most recent period of substance abuse, between thirty-two and just before thirty-three years old. I was feeling like all was lost, and I couldn't handle the degree of the PTSD symptoms—anxiety, fear, recurrent flashbacks, and nightmares—that I was experiencing.

I engaged in trauma therapy and began trying to understand what was happening to me. What was behind all the feelings I was having? Which I had been attributing, primarily, to things that had happened in my adult life. Through the process of trauma therapy, I uncovered that there were roots to my patterns that were traced back to childhood, based on experiences that I had there that were the template for the PTSD that I experienced as an adult.

Through introspective work and talking therapy, I became aware that I felt that I had been abused sexually during my childhood. It was an abstract idea at the beginning, but felt very true. I wasn't sure at all about what had happened. I became very interested in trying to uncover what had transpired during my childhood. I employed a number of different means, including breathwork and EMDR therapy to try to jog what I had at that point, which felt like repressed memories.

I didn't have any success through any of those measures. I did get an idea about one early incident in nursery school, but it didn't seem like it was the thing that would make my life make sense, or what I was searching for. I was referred to do work with MDMA.

At that point, I really felt like traditional therapy wasn't very effective for me. I probably did make some progress when I first initiated it, but it felt like a vicious cycle and something that wasn't a really great fit for me in general. I was very interested when I learned about MDMA. I actually had a memory right around the time I learned about this work. Once, probably five or six years earlier, where I'd been doing MDMA recreationally, I had a flash about my childhood. I didn't really remember it as much as I felt that I should. I wasn't really in a place that was conducive to uncovering any further information. Actually, what I did was, I took a bunch of different drugs and really buried the experience and the information.

It's interesting that it came back to me right around the time that MDMA with a therapeutic focus really came on my radar. That's one of the things that made me very interested in it, as potentially having some value to uncovering locked information.

In my very first session, it took a little while for the medicine itself to work. It took more than one dose. There was a point in the session where the experience went from being very much in my body, having a good feeling in my body, to breaking open heart consciousness, where I had an experience where my heart was strong enough to allow in information that had otherwise been blocked out. It was so powerful that I feel like it just couldn't be processed in ordinary consciousness. I started to physically relive being raped by a school teacher when I was seven years old. The physical experience came first, but I knew very soon after exactly what it was I was remembering, and I continued to physically relive the trauma for an extended period. I had a lot of contractions in my abdomen along with pain and fear. Different emotions were released that had been pent up for, at this point, twenty-nine years.

I realised I had been abused. I realised that there was a hospital-isation that had occurred after the abuse as a result of it, which was something that always didn't make sense in my experience of my childhood. Really, what it felt like was happening was that the medicine allowed for there to be a dialogue between my heart, mind, and soul. It was really like my higher self was able to step in, which was something that I realised I'd been cut off from, and had a download. That was a lot of my experience of PTSD, being cut off from my higher self.

The medicine allowed a mechanism for this information to process through my heart, mind, soul, and higher self, and to begin the long process of integrating what happened and healing from what had been so locked away. In retrospect, I see I was still pretty far from getting this information before I came upon MDMA. It was intense to relive the experience; at the same time, it was also completely doable with the assistance of the MDMA. It was almost like the medicine kept me right at my threshold for re-experiencing this. It didn't give me as much as would break me, but it did give me what I could handle the entire time. This went on probably for an hour or so, maybe two hours tops, and after that point, I had a slowing down of the physical experience, but an ability to begin sorting it out emotionally, to really give context to the way my life had been since the abuse and sort of understand the difficulties that I've experienced throughout life, and troubles, their origins, that prior to now, I didn't even know had happened. Sort of reshuffling the deck a little bit. The medicine was very good for that. It allowed this expanded heart consciousness for me to be able to begin to integrate the information.

A little while after that, the MDMA starts to slowly wear off, and there's definitely a feeling of rawness and vulnerability that was left. And a whole lot of information to process. It's been six years since I did the work itself. It was like the key that I was able to put into a lock that opened up the process of healing and coming to some peace in my life. I've been able to get much better from symptoms of PTSD, although I still do struggle sometimes. Much less severity of symptoms and frequency of episodes. I've done work in other group settings with other survivors of child-hood sexual abuse, and I've found that to be very helpful. I've continued my exploration of working through these events in a non-ordinary state of consciousness by working with various plant medicines from Central and South America that continue to be of great benefit in integrating and healing from traumatic events of my past.

J's path to this work involved various methods to try to gain access to the feelings suggestive of childhood sexual abuse that he was experiencing. Talk therapy, breathwork, EMDR, were all of value but failed to bring him to be able to revisit the event itself, to re-experience it, enabling its release. The psyche needs our involvement in this interactive process, needs to know we are ready to face the personal horror that we have internalised, but of which we may have no knowledge. The psyche, ever on our side, needs this knowledge, the details of the event, in order to know what to do. Once the specifics are known, once the psyche understands that one is in a safe and supported place and that what it has been holding onto is from the past, twenty-nine years in this instance, it releases.

The embrace of the medicine enabled him to revisit, remember, and understand what had happened to him. The medicine creates a buffered distance from the traumatic memory laid bare in the medicine session, making the revisit 'completely doable'. During the subsequent hospitalisation for rectal bleeding, medical professionals examined every possibility of origin for over a week, yet completely ignored the possibility of bleeding from an anal tear caused by the sodomy perpetrated upon this seven-year-old boy. This one violent incident shattered his innocence, and the normal, happy, and wholesome direction of his childhood was over. The self-medication of his subsequent life was pre-ordained by this single, terrible incident that had disfigured his body, mind, and spirit in one fell swoop.

• • •

Going for my first session, I was absolutely filled with fear.

A. Z.

A. Z. approached the work both gingerly and deliberately, following clues in conversations and the experiences of friends. One was the father of an intellectually brilliant young man whose academic career, and indeed his life, had become stalled with severe depression and anxiety. He exposed himself to the medicine, and in one session found the release that has enabled him to successfully complete his studies.

A. Z. is a thoughtful, talkative individual from a distant location whose nervousness had expressed itself at the consultation as well as on the session day. He was naïve to any 'drug' experience but found great value in his sessions, with insights and epiphanies about personal and political matters. He credits the work for giving him increased mindfulness and connection in every moment, enabling the implementation of significant changes in his life.

I was first introduced to the medicine by a friend whose child had exhausted all psychiatric remedies and was in very bad shape.

They had come across it as sleep-deprived insomniacs, searching the internet all night in desperation and became curious. This work eventually helped cure their child, who otherwise had a very bleak prognosis; no psychopharmacological medications were working, and he had been treated at top hospitals and treatment centres. The child went back to college, has now graduated, and lives a normal, full life.

My only prior 'drug' experience, other than pot (which I did inhale at college and very occasionally one or two times a year since), was when I was twenty years old and accidentally took LSD at a rock concert.

Then, another friend, who I would never have expected to be doing anything like this (illegal/weird), outed themselves, and that helped legitimise it.

Finally, another friend who had started 'journeying' was extolling the virtues, learnings, and growth opportunities.

When I started asking around, very carefully and discreetly, I began hearing more stories of people who are involved in 'journeying' and the profound effects. Nobody speaks about it openly, and it is usually the other person broaching the topic, unless the space is deemed to be somehow safe, but then the tremendous learnings occur.

It's a very strange situation. So many are being profoundly, positively affected, and even at major international gatherings at which I have the opportunity to participate on topics of world issues, I serendipitously get involved in conversations once people open up. Unfortunately, I often feel unable to introduce others to the possibilities.

The impact of this stigma is profound as it keeps people from openly sharing, talking on the phone or in emails about their experiences. But it's illegal, as well as alcohol during prohibition, marijuana, homosexuality, harbouring, and helping escaped slaves, blacks using whites-only bathrooms, and a host of other laws now viewed as anachronistic and often immoral. It is very unfortunate they were even there during their time.

This is a valuable, powerful medicine to help those in need, in addition to the 'well,' to expand their own consciousness and life experience. Criminalising it is absurd.

My curiosity finally got the better of me, although I must confess that going for my first session, I was absolutely filled with fear.

In terms of measurable impact on my personal life and ignoring the total spiritual growth and opening, I have become much more generous and compassionate about the suffering of others, and less judgemental about things that had bothered me in those to whom I am closest. I have more compassion for my mother, who is wheelchair bound, as well as for her aides, which 'shocked' my mother by the level of the gratitude gift I gave them, and I think opened new doors and possibilities for her, including impactful change in their relationship with my mother. This was not intentional or manipulative, but it was a wonderful outcome. I also had an experience of imagining completely locked muscles, generating empathy for my mother's immobility.

I had a realisation reliving an incident of driving on a long bridge with my younger siblings when I was ten years old. They briefly (maybe for ten seconds) teased me that we would drive off the bridge into the river below. If one joking-and-teasing comment had a lifelong effect, what had I maybe done by accident, or had otherwise happened to someone else? I have not lived their life experiences and cannot possibly (as in 'I am not able to'), have judgements about others and their 'irrational fears', 'triggers', and 'issues.'

Medicine sessions also helped me extinguish other fears, such as an irrational fear of trucks passing when I am bicycle-riding. (Rational caution is helpful and protective; irrational, paralysing fear is neither.) I experienced a large white truck pulling alongside me and enveloping and protecting me and my bicycle that helped me safely during the cross-country bicycle trip, forever shifting that fear.

I imagined experiencing a very close friend who had experienced early childhood molestation, and I was with him, forever shifting our relationship.

I saw my best friend, who died when we were both twenty-six, as Jesus Christ who sacrificed his body (unintentionally) to teach me life lessons, to enhance my life appreciation and gratitude, and to encourage me to seize and live in the moment.

I am using this only as a very serious medicine and ignoring the 'fun' aspects. It's ironic that I never use it for recreation, which is what it is so known for. I have done a lot of other personal exploration and growth and found in a few medicine sessions tremendously accelerated progress in all dimensions.

After my first session, my wife said I left her the nicest voicemail ever, spoken totally from my open heart, which helped solidify our already wonderful relationship and brought it to better depths.

These sessions have improved my relationship with our children as I am able to be more accepting overall, more open, much more compassionate, and less in fear of them living through their own, sometimes painful, growth experiences, completely suspending judgement.

In the first session, at my request, the attendant took twenty-five pages of notes. I feared that I would miss something if it was not written down. I later realised how my To-Do list obsession and concerns/worries about forgetting kept me from going as deeply as possible into the experience, a great metaphor for my life. I also realised my Outlook Calendar was always packed, and I saw the blocked-out areas as bars on a cage with a few holes for light.

In subsequent sessions, I spoke hardly at all but found that I had a vivid memory of insights (Surprisingly, my memory was more intense and even better than without the medicine).

In a few sessions, I have a much better perspective on my work life too, becoming really tied into purpose and sharing lessons, rather than doing things as achievements, to satisfy others' expectations or so they 'like' me. The effect of turning off the left side of my brain, which is generally dominant and controls everything I do, also helps me in getting rid of so many of the 'shoulds'. I got to what is behind them and that is what I truly want.

While the short-term effect, when the medicine is in the system, is a wonderful feeling of expansiveness and love, it is the long-term changes, the half-life, that I have found to be amazingly impactful. There is a dramatic impact and change in so many areas.

I find myself now living much more from a place of abundance and gratitude, where almost anything is possible. Rather than a state of scarcity, fear and 'shoulds', from this place anything seems possible and 'negative' experiences are viewed as learnings and opportunities in the true sense, rather than perfunctorily.

Judgements have been replaced by opportunities for perception and discernment.

It is bizarre that the war on drugs has created a broad category of different and completely unrelated substances with widely divergent profiles of beneficial impact and potential risks, all of which are subject to prohibition, notwithstanding the fact that besides being ill-advised, the war on drugs does not work and just puts masses of people, primarily minorities, in prison. On the other hand, opioids, which are regularly over-prescribed, (300 million prescriptions in 2015, 80 percent consumed in the US (Source: Dina Gusovsky, CNBC)), are highly addictive and extremely dangerous.

From the place this medicine takes us to, conflict becomes ludicrous, usually about things that do not matter, particularly geopolitical conflicts in the name of one artificially defined group versus another. It gives empathy and compassion for oneself and others, which makes judgements almost impossible. Discernment replaces this from an open and loving place. You become a mini Dalai Lama.

It has huge benefits on an emotional, relational, intellectual, and spiritual level; questions become so much more clearly answered, relationships improve, and a sense of connection to something, whatever that may be for each individual—God, Universe, Spirit within—is created or enhanced.

I find myself seeking greater purpose, higher truth, and deeper and more meaningful interactions with people in general. There is a challenge remembering that whereas I may have been through an experience which has changed me, others I am interacting with have not, so I cannot make assumptions about their openness and receptivity.

Vulnerability is amplified one-hundredfold and one must exercise reasonable boundaries.

Set and setting are critical. This is serious work, not recreational. It is important that dosages and intentions are clear and maintained.

Meditation is always difficult for me with a wonderful but hyperactive monkey-mind. Since beginning the medicine work, I have been able to meditate much more deeply.

Stripping away the intellectual filters brings me to simple and unconditional love, much as we feel pure love for our children and pets.

Intentions are critical. I was very fortunate in not having any serious psychological issues.

I am aware of others who have used this as a last resort with miraculous outcomes, after all regular pharmaceutical drugs and treatment have been unsuccessful. The idea that this must be done 'under the table', with twenty-two veterans in the United States committing suicide every day who might be helped by this medicine, the idea that we are not using all available possible resources, including this medicine's potential, based on preliminary testing results and lab studies, is the greatest disservice to those human beings in our country, our military, and the world at large.

So many insights.

Scheduling sessions between his worldly engagements, A. Z. has achieved most everything his friends had suggested might be possible through exposure to MDMA. His life of conferences, meetings, and public events in various locations continues as he also gives time to his own re-creation. This testimony, gratefully received, was mailed from the Camino De Santiago pilgrimage route in Spain.

• • •

There's always room for improvement.

Andreas.

Andreas was in a fix when he came to the work. None of the strategies that he had developed during his life, since as far back as his childhood were working anymore, but with courage and constancy, he has come to a place where he is at peace with himself. His bad-boy attitude to life was not his true self but the predictable reaction to a confused, brutal, and unloving childhood.

What brought me to the work, what I became unhappy with, was the repetition of certain patterns over and over again. I knew where it came from, but I don't think I was ever able to really get too deep into it, or allow myself to not be strong. All my defence mechanisms were pushing me to avoid breakdown by becoming stronger than ever, which led to a decent amount of aggression. In work environments, if I didn't get things done in certain ways with some of my vendors, I would lose my shit.

I was ready for something different. I could talk about my bad patterns all day long, but I couldn't really feel anything about them. I couldn't get into that healing spot. All the childhood stuff was boxed away, stuffed way, way down. I thought I was bigger and stronger than anything, and that was the whole problem.

The one emotion I allowed was anger. Everyone always made fun of my temper, but in a way, anger seemed normal to me. Growing up in the years that I did, it was pretty violent. I remember I used to get in fights with my father, and then I'd just go out and walk in the evening. At every other house, I'd hear yelling and screaming. You used to just see fights in the street all the time. If a cab driver drove too close to you through an intersection, you punched him through the window. That was just normal behaviour.

I had a very bad temper, and I started getting to an age where I was just like, "This really isn't good." I decided that it was time to really start looking into changing. I started some work with a therapist.

A friend put me on to an attendant and MDMA therapy. I found a cognitive behavioural therapist I still work with, and he's been very helpful, introducing me to meditation and other stuff like that, which has been great. The combination of the two has worked out tremendously.

I'd tried other things before. The last time I went to a therapist was after I got in a little bit of trouble when I was younger, and I had to go away. I owned my business at the time. It was really, really stressful; I threw a computer through a glass desk. The stress was just too much. I was trying to maintain my business while prepping to go to jail for two months, and it became too much for me, so I started to see a therapist.

I also work out and do things like that to get out my aggression, but that wasn't cutting it. I worked a couple times with somebody who teaches Core Energetics, but he was really pricey and insurance didn't cover it. I started reading a lot of New Age pioneer and guru Osho to begin with, and then a little bit of Core Energetics founder Pierrakos, and a lot of stuff, just to get a better feel of certain things. Then, I got a recommendation from somebody who asked, "Okay, are you aware of, say, MDMA as a potential therapeutic tool?"

I had heard about it but never really delved too deep into it. I've known about work here and there, and test studies done a while back. I knew a lot about MDMA itself. I was one of the first arrests made in my county for MDMA after it was put on the calendar.

I had done my share of stuff when I was a kid, but I never got too into any one thing. Before I went to a therapist, I found myself getting a little too caught up with cocaine. I self-medicated with opiates for quite a few years. It was not horrible, but getting messed up every weekend wasn't good for my business. I was like, "Okay, I'm going to be forty soon. I've got to not do this shit anymore."

My problems probably came from growing up with a father who was borderline insane; I knew that. I knew where it came from, and I knew that a lot of my habits weren't acceptable, but still, when you just grow up around it, it's kind of built into you. I watched my father lash out in public at a Sears employee and things like that, causing a huge scene. Because you get used to that type of behaviour, it kind of numbs you to it, so when you do it, you don't see it as such a big deal. Luckily, I've always had a little bit of awareness, going, "That's not really the thing you should be doing."

For a long time, I wouldn't allow myself to say my childhood was that bad, so that was one of the biggest things that I worked through after my MDMA work, allowing myself to say, "You know what, it was bad." I had to talk to my mother and my sister and tell them to stop saying it wasn't that bad. I was like, "If life with my father wasn't that bad, all of us would still be talking to him." None of us have spoken to him in fifteen years.

I had used MDMA before, when I used to go out clubbing, but never for self-reflection. I had no idea what to expect from therapeutic MDMA at all. I was slightly nervous the first time and the second time, I was really worried. I was afraid I was going to find out things I didn't want to know. The fear wasn't debilitating, though.

I went into the MDMA sessions knowing a lot about my issues, particularly with my father, but also realised that I had a lot of hatred for my mother. I'd displaced it, because my father was so crazy. The first session was intended to focus on my father. For the second one, I went in with the intention of dealing with my mother. It went somewhere else, and I had to come back for the third one, to finally break through what happened at the second one.

During my first session, I had a section where I was a little bit paranoid. I got stuck halfway through or something. I was just getting freaked out. I was getting kind of used to it, and I was doing what I call mental gymnastics. I got lost in reality constructs for who knows how many hours. I was thinking, "All right, so what's real? Is me feeling this real?" It's good stuff that I was going through, not 100 percent pertinent to what my issues were, but I think good, in general, because you could see that maybe my father saw something one way and I saw something another way, and he couldn't see what I saw, or something like that. I could apply it to different things afterwards, but during, it was definitely a little bit intense.

In the second session, I realised that I had blocked out a lot of my childhood, so I started going back, seeing some more things I didn't remember. I had to shut off the second session mid-peak. I was coming to something that I didn't want to broach at that moment, and I turned off. I looked up. I was like, "I don't know. I don't really feel anything." I shut it down for at least an hour, took off my eye mask, and left to go home. In the cab, though, the effects came back. I muscled through it and went to bed.

During the next session, I came across it again, and I was fidgeting a lot. My attendant asked if I was all right, and I'm like, "Yeah, I had an image of a black house, and I was just like, 'I'm going to just kind of chill out around the house for a little bit.'" I decided to take a second dose at that point, because the vision was just kind of hanging out there, and that's when the house exploded open. The visual was basically a tornado of shit, and a little dot in the middle, which was me. The shit was my mother and my father swirling around, and there was a little stuck me in the middle of this house.

After that explosion through, I started kind of moving around. I think I had my hand in my mouth, at one point. I was just moving through stuff. It felt like I was almost a newborn on the couch, and I was just moving my arms around, and I was pushing through, and I literally felt like a kid.

That was phenomenal, because I would never flail around on the couch in front of anybody with my hand in my mouth. It's just my self-control. But, there I was, flailing around on the couch like a fool. Even with the flailing, I just felt amazing.

After that breakthrough, I became much more relaxed. The fourth session was just me going back in to check on some things with my father, with maybe some forgiveness and stuff like that. After that, I was able to e-mail my father for the first time.

After my first session, I decided that I was going to start calling around to some of my family members and ask them some questions.

My first call was to my aunt. She said she remembered me sitting at the table, kind of shaking at dinner, because I'd be worrying if my dad was going to yell at me, or smack me, or something like that. Then, she mentioned that she thought that my dad might have been married before. I was just like, "Wait, what?" It turned out to be true. My father was married to his high school sweetheart. They had a son. She killed the son while he was a newborn, under a year. They admitted her to Bellevue, and afterwards, she hung herself there.

I was born a year and a half after that happened. My first instinct was, did my father drive her to do that? Then, the second thought was, obviously, this would all tie into everything being fucking crazy. I remembered all of a sudden that my father wouldn't leave the house, sometimes for four or five days. He would work nights. Sometimes, he'd stay at home. He wouldn't leave the bedroom at all. I remember food flying out the door and having to tiptoe around the house.

I don't know if my father was already depressed, or if his first wife killing herself and their son made him that way. I'm probably never going to know the truth. I think he was already halfway there, anyway, because my grandfather was a bit of a fucking nut, too.

I don't push people to do the same work I've done, but I'm honest about it. Since doing the work, I've come across people who start talking to me about stuff, and I'm just like, "Oh, well this is something that I've done." Some of them I don't think need this kind of work. Some of them just need basic therapy. I do think everybody would benefit from this, but I think it's hard enough just to get people to go to therapy to begin with.

The work continues long after the sessions. You get revelations. You get your feelings of being okay. I think a lot of it is you're able to go back there, and it's okay to visit there again. It's all right now. You're older. Those days are gone. No one's going to hurt you anymore. It breaks down those defence mechanisms and allows you to go back there. Then, you can take that, moving forward.

It takes some maintenance. The work that I do with the attendant is great. The work that I do with my therapist, once a month, now, is still very important. My daily meditation is the most important. Meditation is like flossing. A medicine session is like going to get my teeth cleaned at the dentist to remove that hard-to-get stuff. It's the daily stuff that's going to keep everything the way it's supposed to be.

It all tied in together quite well. The sessions with the attendant tied together with the meditation, I think, to help me drop not only drugs, but cigarettes and alcohol. It all just kind of fell away. I didn't even consciously say, "I'm going to quit." Quitting cigarettes was the biggest one, because I had smoked on and off for so many years. The meditation slowed me down enough to give me the realisation that when I was walking down the street at 8:00 p.m. thinking, "Oh, I want a cigarette" what I really meant was, "It's 8:00 p.m. I normally smoke a cigarette. That's what I want. I just want my habit right now. It has nothing to do with a cigarette."

As for opiates, which I'd used quite a lot, I don't really have the desire. Once in a while, I catch myself thinking about it, but I think it's just a habitual thing, like if I'm under a lot of stress, I'll be like, "Oh, grab a pill." I have some in a drawer that have just been sitting there for years. I don't touch them. I'm just like, "No, dude. You're stressed. Go for a walk. Go do something else."

My anger has improved dramatically. That has a lot to do with the medicine work and meditation, as well. Through the work, you learn different tactics and tricks to get yourself to not go down those roads, or to look at things a bit differently, from different perspectives, to allow you to step back a minute before that kicks in.

The work with MDMA was important and necessary, but it's not a cure-all. If you just go do some sessions and be like, "Oh, I'm fixed," then I think you're a fool. There's a lot more work involved. You don't have to do it through meditation. There's fifty million different ways to get the same results. You could do it in a lot of different things, but I think it's continual. I don't think it ever stops. You have to keep doing it. There's always room for improvement.

That said, MDMA was vital to put me in touch with the stuff that

I wasn't able to get in touch with in traditional therapy. I think that gave me a huge advantage in therapy; things could happen faster. Whereas, to do what I did would've taken probably years in traditional therapy—years upon years upon years—to get there.

It's kind of like cheating a little bit. You could do it through fasting, through meditation, through dervishing, through breathing. You could get yourself in those places. Do you want to spin around in a circle for three hours, or do you just want to take two pills and just get there a little bit faster?

Still, it's not easy. You need to go in there with intentions of what you want to work on. If you're stuck in there, and your mind is doing what it usually does to you, it's not a comfortable thing to do. It's not something fun. On the other hand, I wouldn't say my sessions have not been pleasant. They've been a lot of fucking work, yes. It's literally work. It's a good eight, ten hours of fucking hard-ass shit. It's like getting a deep tissue massage. I get those a lot, because I work out a lot. That's not a nice massage; it hurts!

Since doing the work, I have reached out to my father. I used to think I'd never speak to my father again. I wanted him to pay for his actions. But now, I've opened that door. He did contact me. He seems pretty much the same, but I'm leaving the door open.

My other relationships have changed too. I have a girlfriend I'm very much in love with. I had taken about two years off from dating while I was doing a lot of work on myself. I've learned a lot of things about what I was doing, and how I would self-destruct relationships and things like that. Based on all these things that we were subjected to as we were growing up, I'm in a good spot.

Spiritually, I've started getting into a little bit of Buddhism. The precepts, the basic constructs of it, are great. If you go by a certain teaching, and you go by basic principles, they're amazing. It shows that love beats everything. That's the only thing that you can do, is just love everybody, including yourself first. Just remember to smile when you're walking down the street. Life's pretty good, because you're fucking alive, and you're breathing. You've got food. You've got a roof over your head. You have everything in the world to be happy for, you know? Not to downplay any of the damage that you've experienced, but that was a long time ago. It's not like that anymore, so you have to stop living like you're still there.

I think everybody should do this work.

I hope this message gets out there, and I hope it really does get people to start looking at this a little bit more. People need it. I feel connected to everything now. I know we're part of a more expansive universe. I believe that there's other life out there. I believe in stuff outside of our physical realm. I don't need to see that, but maybe some people are so stuck in this world that they do need to see something like that. MDMA, therapy, meditation, and there you are. For so many of us, it's that simple.

I really think that a lot of people need this, and I think that it's really, really bad that it's not accessible to a lot of people. I figured everyone could hide their faces, but I want it to be out in the open. Even with priors related to MDMA on my record, I thought it was important to speak out. Let people see a face and see that it's not too much off the deep end. I think it's good to start seeing normal people, just everyday people, doing stuff like this. I think that was why I thought it was important to tell my story.

Andreas's entire childhood was so traumatic that he had blocked out 'whole chunks' of it, but by staying with the memories as they emerged, he was able to recall and process much of the relentless negativity. One whole chunk was deliberately omitted, salient facts about his father that his family, arguably acting protectively, sought to keep from him. One can only imagine what it was like for him to find out the truth. Finding himself in-session as 'little stuck me in the middle of the house', he expressed this bind by 'flailing around on the couch' that felt 'amazing', and emerged to be able to contact his father for the first time in many years. He used the medicine sessions not as an end in themselves but as way-stations, clearing his path to mindfully engage with his considerable life issues going forward. His experience of the ongoing nature of this work leads him to concur with Stan Grof who has opined, "There is no graduation," and his advocacy of work with MDMA comes from his gratitude for the self-understanding and healing he has experienced. He's "in a good spot."

●　●　●

I was suicidal most of the time, and I just wanted to get out of pain.

Edward G.

Edward came through channels, and our Thursday afternoon consultation ended with him leaving in a huff. I left him alone on Friday but texted him on Saturday and Sunday to let him know I was available for the session day we had arranged for Monday. Getting no response, I could only assume he was no longer interested and made an appointment with a nearby mobility therapist at 11:00 a.m., the time when we would have met. Leaving my house that morning, there was Edward in the driveway, all ready. I said I was surprised to see him, and he said, "It's my Asperger's," at which point I understood that his behaviour was an artefact of this condition and invited him to walk with me to my one-hour appointment. We talked fruitfully, and he expressed that he was ready to work, so we met at noon for his first session.

I was in my mid-twenties, and my life was a bit of a mess. I'd had bad depression my entire life with periods of it getting better and then periods of it getting worse. I was at an all-time low. I had a lovely wife (I still have a lovely wife). Other than that, I struggled with relationships, working on a business project and failing, and just completely shutting down as a person. My depression would come out as physical pain, confusion, loss of focus. My desire to sleep was just unquenchable. I was suicidal most of the time, and I just wanted to get out of pain.

I had anhedonia, which is where you just don't enjoy anything. My life was a Kafkaesque series of doing things I hoped to enjoy. I did them, didn't enjoy them, and ended up more miserable than when I started. The problems kept multiplying. I was dragging my wife down along with me, because it's incredibly painful to watch, and it was very hard on her, seeing someone she loved in that bad of a shape not being able to help me.

I was helped by stimulants years before. Provigil and Adderall also had beneficial effects. It stopped working. I would still have energy, but it would take me to a very dark place and make me aggressive. It also made the suicidal feelings worse. I stopped doing that and went years without being medicated when this just started getting worse and worse. Before that though, as a teenager, I'd taken about a dozen antidepressants, prescription antidepressants, and SAM-e over the counter.

Asperger's Syndrome was diagnosed in early childhood. Things would be sensory overload. It's like when you see videos of the autistic kid screaming and flapping his hands. I slapped my hands and kicked, things like that. To some degree, I grew out of it, but one of the biggest problems is that autism, almost universally, is accompanied by something called alexithymia, which is the inability to know what you're feeling emotionally. The biggest problem with that is if you deconstruct a human relationship, at the end of it, you don't have much. It looks like either I'm in control, the other person's in control, or our relationship is superficial. This causes obvious problems. There were social aspects beyond missing social cues that came from a rather distorted view of what things were supposed to be like socially.

Someone suggested MDMA therapy, so I looked into it and tried it out. I was in the middle of a hideous time due to some social things I got into. I had trouble with the attendant I met for the consultation. Once I mentioned the Asperger's, it was easier.

At the beginning of the MDMA session, I had what was later described as a most extreme reaction. I very quickly, after taking it, started feeling hideous anxiety, and the attendant said, "Relax into your anxiety," for which I'm still slightly bitter. That was the last adult emotion that I felt. After that, I was screaming through the entire thing. On and off, coming in waves with just pain that I couldn't control. It was an emotional pain. It wasn't anything that could be experienced by an adult, because with an adult, there would be some type of commentary, some type of understanding, some type of mastery, and none of it was there. It was infantile screaming that was me tensing from the stomach in a way that it almost looked like going into the fetal position. Screaming.

Afterward, I felt my ability to feel things better. I had more empathy for other people, and I understood myself a bit better. The effects, the more direct depression effects, were not long-lasting. The emotional insights were, but I did end up having to go back and go through it again. My second session was almost identical to the first, except that they had made the treatment room considerably more indestructible, because I was all over it screaming, not particularly in control. After that, it was a similar result. Some more temporary relief, plus some long-term insights.

There were many different causes, and things became apparent using different modalities over different periods of time. By doing the medicine work over and over, I was able to get a better understanding of myself and had some mental improvement, if not psychiatric improvement.

Edward's first session was every bit as violent as he describes, and I feared for the integrity of the couch; hence the attention to the treatment room for subsequent sessions. He is a big chap, and the tremendous energy he expressed as convulsions continued for hours and hours. Follow-up sessions saw him literally all over the room, throwing cushions like a child having a tantrum, leading eventually to sessions where, for substantial periods of time, he was ruminating within in relative stillness. He has subsequently found out from inquiries within his family that, when he was an infant, his older siblings would delight in tickling him and tickling and tickling him, until they were done with it; there was no restraint from his parents. It would be over-reaching to suggest a direct link between these events of Edward's infancy to his longstanding diagnosis of Asperger's, but in our view attention should be paid.

* * *

Our wisdom to move toward wholeness is innate.

Mark M.

Childhood sexual abuse signals the end of innocence for the victim, and this loss endures indefinitely as an ongoing existential threat. In an instant, we understand that we are no longer inviolable. The event or events rob us of our natural developmental ability to become ourselves; our essential 'being' now compromised by the real possibility of a trifecta of threat; at any time, in any place and by any person. The complexity of feelings that arise, only to be suppressed, are a mosh-pit of conflicting emotions, beliefs, hopes, and fears that can leave the victim greatly challenged in developing their own unique identity. Ongoing attempts to do so during adulthood may be thwarted from misreading the often-distorted information floating around in one's psyche.

Through many years of talk therapy, I finally came to admit and to understand that the sexual abuse I experienced as a child growing up in a Catholic and alcoholic home left me in the grip of PTSD. I struggled with suicidal impulses, anxiety, and depression. With great effort and a lot of work through my adult years—meditation, yoga, continued talk therapy and creative writing—by the time I was fifty years old, I had reached a place of fairly steady health, and along with the continued bouts of anxiety and depression, relative peace. I'd been blessed after all with a good life, working as an actor and writer and living many years with a loving husband.

But at the age of fifty-five, I tumbled into the fiercest depression I had ever known. It was triggered by a sudden professional disappointment—being let go from a beloved job. I understood it was just business, a frequent hazard in my line of work, but I was utterly dismantled. Profound and painful feelings of failure and utter self-loathing seized me. I couldn't sleep. For several months, I moved through a fog of grief. I intuited that this pain had to do with something larger, more ancient, than the loss of this single job. I was despondent, thinking: "Jesus, am I back to square one? Back to the days of suicidal despair? Have I not, after all these years, got to the bottom of my 'stuff?'"

I realised, that once again, I had to find help. Furthermore, I concluded that the time had finally come to "give in" and seek medical intervention in the form of antidepressants. In the course of seeking advice from various health professionals, the use of MDMA in relation to trauma was mentioned to me. I felt resistance and fear around this idea. But, at the same time, a deep intuition and genuine curiosity led me to meet with a counsellor, an older man, who I learned had extensive training and experience working with this medicine.

During my initial consultation, I described the state I was in. We talked at length about how the trauma I'd experienced long ago was making itself known again at this late stage; at a time when I had less of the basic youthful grit to simply stuff it down and soldier on. The core of the trauma was still there and hankering to be examined again. Yearning, in fact, to finally *get off stage,* as he put it. Many aspects of our conversation resonated with me. By the time our meeting was done, I felt moved to try this approach. I knew I wanted to explore the raw feelings, at least give this method a try, before turning to a pharmaceutical path that would be based more, it seemed to me, on suppressing my feelings.

I would need many pages, I think, to describe fully the ensuing experience, but I want to attempt to capture with some concision how profoundly and positively this work affected me, and how it remains vivid and immensely helpful to this very moment.

It was a fine spring morning when I arrived for my session. I was very nervous. My attendant set me at ease. It was amazing to think that he had blocked off his entire day. He made it clear that the session itself would last for several hours, and in addition, there was no exact limit on our time. If I needed to remain and rest well into the evening, it would be fine with him. The sense of being 'on the clock' vanished, and the generosity of this meant a great deal to me.

The session took place in a warm, beautifully decorated home. There were many natural objects—sea shells, stones, and lovely decorations. The room, for me, somehow thrummed with a calming sense of a connection to the earth, to history. I lay on a comfortable couch. A blanket and sheets were there, if needed (I did eventually end up curling, gratefully, under the sheets). My attendant explained that he was there for anything I might need, but also relayed that he would remain quiet and allow me and the medicine to 'do the work.' I appreciated that: No call to speak, to engage, unless I truly wished to. He indicated that he would jot down notes of anything I happened to say, so I could have them for future reference (To this day, I keep those notes near at hand). With a glass of orange juice, I swallowed my dose, put on a sleeping mask, and lay back. Soothing music, mostly Handel, initially played. The music, which was varied throughout the session, aided me immensely, accompanying and abetting an inward journey.

At some point, well into the first hour, I noticed a change in my body and being. A sense of warmth, of vibration. What I recall most vividly was the feeling of being cradled. As if being embraced, rocked in a small, warm boat that was flowing down a river to a cavern at once within me and beyond 'me.' A cavern that, I sensed, rested at the heart of the matter. As time went on, I knew I was entering what I, myself, labelled 'dark' territory. But the feeling of safety, the cradling, *never* left me. The presence of my attendant sitting quietly across the room was also a vital part of the sense of trust and safety I felt throughout.

I began to feel powerful emotions in my body. I have been a dancer most of my life, and I felt the urge, the need to move. I got to my knees and bent forward and backwards, as if wrestling through bone and muscle, wrestling with memory. I began to cry out, to feel and hear the strength of my voice. This seemed important, somehow, *to find voice.* It was as though I was locating the cry I stifled as a kid. With that continuing sense of safety, I entered into a place (I picture it as a dark mass, an energy field deep within my belly but at the same time somehow...infinite) that had to do with my initial trauma—the very first time, shortly after my twelfth birthday, that I was taken up to an attic at a boy's summer camp and molested.

It was as if a pure rage, a self-caring rage, that I had sought all my life, was being uncovered, released. Rage that a man, two decades my senior, turned me into his sexual toy when I was a prepubescent child. It was as if I could feel back to my hairless body, the very tissue of the little boy who knew *nothing* of sex, had never had an orgasm. I had thought about and worked intellectually for years to analyse and understand this complex event in my life: The terror, the pleasure, the confusion of that sexual entanglement, which began that night and endured until I was nearly sixteen years old. But suddenly, working with the medicine, it was as though I'd entered a gateway to truly *FEEL* it.

"NO, NO. Stop! *This is not my choosing!*" I shouted; I cried it out loud! Remarkably, in all my years of therapeutic work, I had never actually said this aloud! Never yelled like this. It was terrifying and thrilling. I felt a terrific permission and safety to enter into the very core of the memory. What I touched was the sheer and utter kid-panic. I could feel it, for the first time, crying up from my tissue: I AM A LITTLE KID! THIS IS NOT MY FAULT!

This was and remains a crystal clear moment, a sense of having grasped, viscerally, the violence upon my nervous system. And I am someone who from the time, in my mid-thirties, that I uncovered the memories and extent of the abuse, has been at work on this stuff. Now, curled on that couch, at fifty-five years old—yelling—I knew I was uncovering a profound piece, a shard in my belly that I had only vaguely sensed was there and craving air. All my life, I have been embarrassed that I did not *say out loud* what I felt at the time which was: "Wait! Wait. I am not ready for this." How many times had I written or spoken about knowing that the molestation and ensuing abuse was not MY doing. I intellectually understood that. But here it was, the gift (and it was a gift!) of FEELING the panic, the shutdown, in short: *The trauma.*

It was as if I had been looking for this all my life. To understand why, in fact, other people called what happened to me "traumatic." This was something I could never quite accept, always hearing an unkind, untrue voice in my head, saying, "You were not a soldier in Vietnam. You were not a witness to murder. This was sex, and you were a little budding homosexual, after all. Weren't you just asking for it?" A part of me wanted to be touched; it felt good. How dare you compare the terror of battle with being molested as a child—a lonely, curious child. It was as if I finally viscerally *understood* how, through all these years, I could never justify, allow for the truth, the reality, the terror, of my own trauma.

My molester didn't, after all, sodomise me, so, OK, this was no big deal. But here, at last, was the clarity of feeling how violent the whole experience (especially the fact that I had my very first orgasm the night I was initially molested) and relationship was to my body, psyche, and spirit. I needed to understand just how frightening it was and how much that boy, and now this man, had to cope with from that moment on, to continue to live within that Catholic community and beyond it.

In the session, even right at the moment of screaming out (and the ensuing days), I could feel my very soul saying, "Thank you. Thank you! You see now what you endured? What happened? So, go easy on yourself, man. You're a good man, and you're doing well. You are not an evil piece of shit loser who allowed yourself to get molested because you wanted it. You were a kid. Period."

On some level, this may sound simple. But what the medicine gave me was a deep sense of compassion and a basic understanding of the root of my self-hatred. Glimpsing and feeling my little boy confusion, in all its authenticity, gave way to floodgates of love. It took days, several weeks even, to integrate the intensity of this session, but what came over me was a sense of well-being. This sense of deep tenderness toward the man, the soul, I am. Quelling the inner voices that so habitually denigrate my sacred being. I was able—more than four decades after the abuse began—to acknowledge what I had suffered and endured. And with this deep acknowledgement came renewed waves of love and respect. It released a seismic sort of pain and energy that felt literally locked in my belly. And continues to unlock.

Many difficult feelings came up. The tears flowed and with them came waves of liberation from, to put it simply, the self-hatred that plagued me. A deep gratitude arose. As if the child within was saying, "Thank you. Thank you for understanding what I endured. Do you see now, dear man, what a good person you are? You did your best; you were there living life, and we did what we had to do to keep on. Thank you for taking the time to feel and see and breathe through what we breathed through then, so many years ago."

And during the journey on the couch, there was a continuous dialogue with an inner teacher, infinitely wise, connected to deepest self, indeed, to the infinite empathy and compassion that rests at the centre of existence. Woven in the wisdom of the body, this persistent sense of being cradled within the much larger context of simply being human, being alive.

I recall walking home after that first session and seeing a Hasidic man on the street, coming out of temple. He had a prayer book, wearing the very traditional orthodox garb. I said hello to him. Our eyes met. And oh, oh, the love I felt (still do), thinking, yes, here we are; here you and I are, sharing this human moment. I had such a wave of feeling how unlocking compassion for myself, my own 'story,' was a doorway to human compassion.

I decided to do two more sessions over the course of the next five months.

The second two sessions were quieter and even deeper than the first. I felt called to trust stillness, to lie back and accept the journey and the medicine as more of a meditation. These sessions, while still touching upon the childhood sexual trauma, gave rise to more 'material' and memories of my nuclear family. Memories of early childhood, even birth, emerged as an exploration of landing in the troubled home of an alcoholic dad and a suicidal mother. I was being led, it seemed, to a deeper understanding of the context of being an unsupervised, lonely, and curious kid—a target for molestation. This territory was not easy to visit. Painful and sad but in the cradle of the medicine, there was a larger sense of compassion for my parents and their history, *their* struggles. As if grasping the ancestral hum of an ongoing story of working out pain, waking to awareness.

In these two final sessions, I journeyed deeper to the root of what I would call my feelings of "badness." Of being, essentially, 'evil' somehow. I allowed the feelings to come, to enter into this darkness that I had carried for a lifetime. I experienced a surprising physical reaction: A kind of peristaltic, dry vomiting, an almost monstrous sounding expiation of the sense of 'badness' cauterised in my belly. At one point, I actually pictured a 'demon' there deep in my belly with fangs, serpent-like, challenging me to face it, face the darkness and to see "it" as a story, an illusion? My attendant was acutely and physically present at these moments, quietly supporting me, holding a bucket, as I "got it out!"—a kind of bile from way down within flesh and memory. Deep relief followed. I lay back, in peace. Not fully understanding the mystery of what I'd been guided to uncover, expel, but feeling nonetheless a great sense of cleansing.

The integration of these powerful sessions and daily practice of being an aware human being continue, *of course*. Challenges remain. But my gratitude to the medicine and to my calm attendant is boundless. I have no question that the fundamental insights I was given through this work will continue to unfold. The words "heal" and "whole" come from the same root. This medicine is a healer. It has reminded me just how wise, at the deepest level of our being, we are. *I am.* Our wisdom to move toward wholeness is innate. And I continue to believe that the trauma I experienced has been, in a profound and mysterious way, a doorway to the wholeness of this self. To a life lived more fully.

It is my hope that others who are seeking help with trauma are able to find their way to this healing, and I dare say, holy work.

This individual's experiences speak to the psychic complexity resulting from traumas, especially sexual traumas experienced during our development, and to the difficulties inherent in resolving them. Our developing body literally grows upon the already traumatised body, cell by cell, each believing this to be normative. It is not. Additionally, any experience of trauma in childhood rewires the circuitry of the brain and leads it to misinform aspects of our life, inexorably bringing us to the belief that we ourselves are damaged and, in Mark's case, even 'evil.' We are not. The corrective experience available to us under the benevolent influence of MDMA can result in the release of these distorted beliefs and restore us to a more wholesome and balanced appreciation of who we really are.

* * *

The mind is a torrential tyrant.

Anonymous Seeker.

A certain bias is revealed by our self-description, Homo sapiens, namely our fealty to the primacy of our considerable cognitive capacities; I think, therefore I am. This is true, but our obeisance to such an incomplete descriptor allows us to believe that our capacity to think is boundless and we can figure our way out of any problem. This seeker had followed that path, only to find himself getting some understanding in talk therapy but essentially spinning his wheels with regard to the incoherent darkness that lived at his core. Non-ordinary consciousness researcher Stan Grof has often expressed, "If the mind was capable of healing itself, it would have done so a long time ago," and the experiences described in the following testimony radically support that contention.

In a spiritual quest for increased awareness, I was falling into a void of darkness when the mystery and inexplicable wonder of being were thrust upon me. The conundrum of "getting out of the mind" is that every attempt appears to provide the illusion of escape, but only intensifies the labyrinth of horror that the mind has so easily created. The mind is a torrential tyrant in its capacity to control and hold what it thinks to be true, and as a result of the trauma I experienced as a young child, the whole matter of trusting has been difficult. I also see how PTSD has played a significant role in keeping my mind ensnared in an entangled web of survival. I am only now experiencing the shock and fallout of trauma that occurred years ago. I see how it was necessary at a young age to vacate my body, to [enter] extreme dissociated states of mind in order to survive. One doesn't recognise the extent of dissociation one inhabits until one is given an opportunity to witness it from a higher, if not more embracing, perspective. This rare point of view was given to me vis-à-vis this medicine work.

When I came to the couch, I came through insufferable grievances aggravated upon a traumatic past. However, through time, I have seen that trauma can be a doorway to a passageway that leads beyond suffering, on the other side of a fragmented self. I once had a dream that indicated that going through the eye of the needle was tricky—doable, but tricky—and it was through this doorway that I could find freedom from the sexual trauma that has plagued me for most of my life. It is easy to say, "Just let it go," but to let go of the only thing you know is frightening takes considerable courage, if not a great deal of trust, to be pretty sure that in giving up control one will be safe. But there is no definite way of holding onto that idea of what is "safe," because one may never have been safe in the first place. The medicine work allows for the extravagant giving up of one's ego to experience an opening of the heart chakra and its benevolent, amazing beauty. I am uncertain to date where I would be, if I hadn't discovered this blessing.

In my first medicine work session, the sensation of astonishing opening was alarming, to the degree that I witnessed an increasing resistance to an exceedingly greater perspective of being. I was offered an intense capacity to feel. There was incredible excitement in the air. Doorways opened, and the constriction in my chest rose with incredible intensity—the trauma held in the heart cavity heightened to such a degree, my back arched higher, and then the whole matter collapsed, falling back to the couch. I was inside the realm of the heart. My mind had let go, had given up its control and I was free. For once, I felt safe; for once, I was deep within my heart and body and felt like a child; I was home. The state of deep ease created a unity of being between the traumatic memories of my mind's past to the transformation of the present moment. I was breathing alive; I was vibrant and without fear. No division of time was possible. I existed, and the latent idea of fear, the terror of being abused, had subsided. I was breath, and I was being, a universal "me."

During one session, I remember falling into a sudden possession of my body, and the attendant noted it and allowed me to become aware of it. The experience was distinctly foreign. I became aware of the degree of dissociation that I was living out of. I didn't know any better. In that instant, I was able to see walls of glassed hallways interlaced with mirrored doorways that offered no escape. This allowed for little room or freedom to experiment, because my ego self was fragmented in those innumerable hallways, fighting to get out, to encumber a thought process that couldn't support my endeavour to become whole, forever waking up and recognising that getting out was to some degree a formidable impossibility. The journey home was complex, and the more I tried to get out, to wake up from the inherent nightmare of feeling split off, the more I entrenched myself in those insufferable glass hallways, battling to get free.

The inner conflict was amplified by grinding my teeth. I could not understand the implications of the conflicted, torn subject matter that resided deep within the realms of my psyche. Some mornings I awoke with raging jaw pain and headaches from an extensive night of grinding, working through the trauma from the past. The mind is a miracle of divine invention, and it is also a nightmare of its own human complexity and deception. The power of the mind has the capacity to convince beyond a doubt that the traumatic event never occurred. One doesn't want to face the truth and its inherent suffering, of having to come face-to-face with an isolated reality that a loved one forced a violent assault upon a young, trusting child. The matter remains consequential beyond doubt. Innocence and love were rampaged in that infraction. The grace and innocence of a young child were raped, torn from being adored and accepted in purity, and love was forever tempered with distrust and betrayal.

On the couch, I discovered that this medicine work allowed me to lay down this persistent grinding and for a few hours to retreat from the invasion of abuse. It was to be gifted with a perception of a greater possibility of the mind being in unison with heart and body, and not forever lost in its evolving labyrinth. It gave me a chance to relax, gave my mind an opportunity to be calm, to reflect, and see its peril, the persistent fighting to survive and figure out its own conundrum to be free of the antagonistic nature of trauma. It gave an undeniable opportunity to see realities exist beyond the mayhem of mind, in its futile attempts to free itself from a dissociated, traumatic infraction.

Once, I had the pleasure of visiting a psychiatrist's office, and after a brief disclosure of past events, he told me in blatant honesty, "You've got disorder of the self, usually, but not necessarily, caused by childhood trauma, and there's nothing I can do about it." I was out the door within fifteen minutes, walking in hunched dissatisfaction for I had fallen into abysmal depths of confusion, a disarray of enhanced misunderstanding, pounding down upon the concrete, and at one point, in the movement of walking south on a busy, car-ridden street, I accepted that I couldn't fall any further down, so to lick the pavement of that doctor's disgustingly relevant prognosis.

Denial is a powerful absurdity. I was in a deep, disturbing sleep about the past; a contorted distaste of shame lay at the core of my deceived, disenchanted childhood, and the guilt of a shameful act was choked back at the expense of self. I lay obliterated from the impact of dishonesty and was sleepwalking in a coma of amorous disgust. It was too difficult to face the inexorable fact that my father had abused me, and it didn't make sense. I went to a friend's spiritual church and was invited to consider that I had been in an insufferable denial about my past and its consequences.

I am uncertain if the reader has had experiences of waking up in the nightmare of trauma, a constant declaration that one's life has been lived in a deep, perpetual trance. In rendering all emotional, mental, and physical abuses that were subjected upon me in the past, then, and only then, could I begin to perceive how horribly absent I was to the present moment, and to my abusive upbringing. The awakening has nothing to do with blame, but no excuse exists to abuse a child, whether at birth or later in youth through a malfunction of sexual intemperance.

Immediately after I was born, I was put into an incubator. I cannot help but imagine the horror of being "tossed" into a Plexiglas box in order to breathe. I am only beginning to understand that the ramifications of trusting these tender sensations that I have experienced on the couch during medicine work, which cannot be manipulated nor denied. It took a long time to accept that I was abused as a child. I spent years in psychoactive denial, although it was evident through revelatory dreams of a fractured, abusive past that I couldn't ignore. The purity of witnessing in-session the imprint of trauma flowing through my sphere of vision was beyond words, pure and valid and unquestionable, because in that moment no division of mind was conceivable, no lies were forced to swallow, and the indisputable wonder of being was undeniable.

The medicine work is beyond cognitive understanding, and it is a matter of humble surrendering. I have sensed a psychic split persisting at the core centre of my being. What is a psychic split, and how does it impact one's existence? When I was eighteen years old, I remember being stopped in motion, crossing the bedroom floor, and my psyche cracked open, wider than I had ever experienced, and the wonder of information flooded my mind—it was phenomenal, and everything after that point changed. I saw directly into the superficiality of life, of my family's perceptions of a limited reality, and the lack of its capacity to explain the multiplicity and mystical wonder of the universe. I knew more knowledge existed beyond hard work and toil. I now realise that it wasn't the first time that this split had occurred. This wasn't the first time, since I experienced in medicine work that the first time was when I was born and placed in an incubator.

The matter isn't linear, isn't in the least assimilated through cognitive processes, and that's why the journey is complex and forever enraptured in endless revelations, layering upon layers of consciousness. It is unlike any experience that can be rationalised in traditional cognitive therapy. Giving up control of the mind actually enhances the capacity of the mind to perceive on multiple levels of existence at one time, the heart cracks open and speaks volumes of poetic, white truth. For an individual who has spent years cultivating the razor-sharp edge of an acute intellect, a mystical breakthrough demands immediate attention. As human beings, the multiplicity of our existence far exceeds the capacity of our intellects to comprehend the infinite range of human consciousness. From my experience, the depth and capacity of the heart to discern truth far exceeds the limited and foreshortened version created by traumatic events, fearfully restricting any expression of pure self-worth.

To be frank, the battle continues to process the shame induced from sexual abuse, the better to alleviate its distortions in those frightening, darkened hallways that know no exit. From my experience, this medicine work allows one to perceive beyond the great depths of trauma and its dissociations, but it remains within the perceiver's choice whether or not to change central, core beliefs. The individual needs to make a conscious decision to work through trauma and reconcile and absolve the abhorrent distaste of an abusive past. It appears to be a desolate matter of heart, and I am in honesty seeking a deeper resolution beyond the mere absolution of disgust.

I wish to be assured that my soul could embrace a divine position of sanctity, forever encompassing compassion and the purity of love. To allow my humble gratitude to spill over without hesitation, within the enormity of distress that has been alleviated through this gracious work and allow the generosity of this passionate and dignified sitter to be recognised, I would lay down my grievous torment and cry innocence upon my mother's lap.

The torturous intellectual path this seeker had pursued for lack of any other viable option is evident in the circumlocution of his prose; the endless efforts of his mind to find solace from a life derailed at birth and forever afterwards. Everything was going according to nature's plan, but his birthing was infringed upon with surgical incision; the labour was forced, and the whole natural process was mechanistically demolished. These interventions resulted in the infant being consigned to an incubator for the first two and a half weeks of his life. His career as an actor was impaired by frequent episodes of 'whiteout,' a loss of connection, a specific dissociation that inhibited his ability to be in character, caused by the multiple infractions of the emotional arrest he had experienced. He expresses the trauma of this sudden separation with a classic understatement, "It was necessary at a young age to vacate my body," but from his consistent work with MDMA, he has been able to begin to feel more fully embodied.

• • •

That body, it's crying out; it's telling you something.

Fearless A.

Fearless was completely naïve about the medicine work, but once he had heard of its potential, he had conducted extensive research online. He came for a consultation on behalf of his wife, whose post-partum depression that she had experienced following the birth of their youngest son had not abated after many years. They had met in high school and Fearless was devastated, saying, "The person I married does not exist anymore." He then brought her to a consultation, and it was agreed that they would do the work together. She took to the work like a duck to water, and they left soon after, against advice, as happy as clams. They subsequently went on vacation, and the whole thing fell apart, resulting in their eventual divorce.

Before MDMA, I was an absolute train wreck disaster. Can't describe it actually, before. Can't even describe it. I was a robot just with my head down, just trying to do things to perhaps even avoid looking at myself. I came to the work to help my spouse at the time, who was struggling with depression and alcohol, and I thought it would be beneficial for us, or significantly beneficial for her. What happened was it was the most beneficial for me.

The only reason I did it was for her, to make her comfortable to do it. I didn't expect any results on myself, but doing it the first time with her and then subsequent times for myself, I was amazed with the power of the work. The simple truth is that nobody knows yourself better than yourself, and your answer lies within.

Who better to fix your problems than yourself? It's just being able to identify yourself, and the medicine gives you the compassion, the higher level of intellect, the entire tools of the toolbox, so you can really look at yourself from a number of different perspectives, understand yourself and other people better. I was in search of something for many years, maybe ten years, before I came to the work, but always depressed, always unhappy, and through the work—and it is work, believe it or not, it's a heck of a lot of work—kind of released me.

There were other modalities that I tried, but if I had to pick the one that was the most successful to get me on the right path and through this journey it was this work. Best way I can describe, my life was always like a jigsaw puzzle—a thousand pieces on the floor. I knew what was wrong with every piece, I just couldn't put it all together. The work finally helped me put it all together.

At first, I thought the work was going to be a tool for somebody else, and then the second time I did the work was to help me relieve some pain, again, that I thought was caused, perhaps, by somebody else, but ultimately, I found that it was all within me. I was the source of all the trouble, source of all the problems.

It's not a painless process, but you grow a lot from your pain, and you don't have to suffer over it. You can release it, you can understand it, and you can understand the purpose for it. Sometimes, there's a purpose for the pain to help you find yourself. You need some impetus to being sick and tired of being sick and tired.

I had a tremendous amount of anxiety. Tremendous amount. One of the simple things and one of the most unsettling things for me was not being able to be still with myself, thinking something was wrong. It was crazy. My whole life just living at 100 or 1,000 miles per hour, because I didn't want to slow down and really look at myself and see who I was. The medicine gave me that opportunity to say, "This isn't who you want to be. This is who you are, so you have to make some behavioural changes to be that person." Instead of it being a drama or a soap opera life, you can start living.

Buttons that would have been pressed before are not pressed anymore, or they press the buttons, and it just doesn't ring the bell. That trigger's broken. Something that would trigger you in the past, it can no longer touch it, because you just won't allow it.

I didn't understand it until later. I knew it was something. I couldn't put my finger on it, and I did do conventional therapy as well, which helped a lot. Once I had done this work, I was able to accept the talk therapy in a much different manner than I was ever able to. Before, they were just words. They were just someone reading out of a book. Nothing stuck, but through exposure to the medicine work, it helped me see that the mind is a very, very complicated tool. Many times, we're just deceiving ourselves and allowing ourselves to stay and live in this pain for whatever label we put on it. Depression, co-dependency, it doesn't matter.

I think the beauty of the work, one of the most important parts of the work, is that it wasn't tainted. It was me in a room with some music and nobody there directing me. I was directing myself. I think there's significant importance of that, that there's no influence from outside. I, personally, found it rewarding to record the session, so I could hear myself. Many times that kept me on track, but I think there's something very authentic and pure about it not being influenced whatsoever and just being yourself.

You're having a meeting with a mind, but you want to have a meeting with your mind, not somebody else's interpretation of your mind. To me, that is of significant importance.

Understanding from the intellectual level is one thing, but then feeling the emotion part is something else. You get an understanding that they're separate, and they're both okay. There's a battle within the mind of judging these feelings, "Why am I feeling?" The torture you put upon yourself for not understanding what they are, I consider it the intellect and emotional part connecting somehow with the core, your centre-self.

That body, it's crying out; it's telling you something. It's happening for a reason. You need to listen to both. Many of us don't; many of us just listen to our minds, and many of us are so afraid to get in touch with those emotions because that could be weakness, but it's telling you what to do; you just need to listen. You just need to listen to yourself. The answer definitely lies within.

The jigsaw pieces that were scattered all over the floor before, now it's a beautiful mosaic, the jigsaw puzzle, when it's put together. That doesn't mean that as I go through life, I might not drop a few pieces here or there. It's a mobile jigsaw puzzle. Without the medicine, I don't think I would ever have the capacity to work, to get to where I am, and I wish I had it when I was fifteen years old. It would have saved thirty years of torture for myself.

It needs to be known. It needs to be known. If I think about the number of doctors and therapists, that either myself or my spouse went to, and everyone wants to just mask the problem with a medicine. Put a Band-Aid on it and pretend it doesn't exist. Well, it doesn't go away that way. It just creates another problem and then another problem and then an addiction problem.

The answer is really simple: The medicine allows you to get in touch with your emotions, understand from an intellectual level what is going on and make that mind-body connection. It'll give you a roadmap. Then, it's up to you what you do with it. Your work starts there, at the end of the session, but it doesn't end there.

You can't just say, "Hey, I'm fixed." It's not that, but it's understanding both mind and body, and now you have a beautiful roadmap in front of you. We all got to do a little work to stay on the path. Sometimes, we're all going to travel a little astray, but once you experience that once, from the medicine, you'll be centred much more. You can't go too far off the path. All of a sudden, if you're off track, you remember back, "Wait, when I did the work," and you're like, "Wow," you can start telling yourself, "Never again." Our minds are very devious. They'll do anything to not let you see the truth.

You can't separate it; you just cannot separate it and just look at it from an intellectual level. That's impossible. I don't know anybody who's more of an over-thinker than I am. I thought

I could think my way out of any problem. All you're doing is putting yourself on a hamster wheel, chasing your own tail like a little dog. This gives you an opportunity to get off the wheel.

We think we're getting close to resolving our problems, and then we'll do it again. It's just a vicious cycle where this thing... It almost allows you to see a little videotape of yourself being that hamster, and you're like, "Oh, my God, I did that for this reason. Oh, my God, I did that for this." Then, it's realising, "Okay, what am I doing now? Am I repeating that past behaviour in a different manner and pretending I'm better, or am I really, really looking at myself?"

Frequently, that's what we're doing. We're repeating these patterns with which we have brainwashed ourselves (or with the assistance of dysfunctional family or whatever, it doesn't really matter), but we continue to repeat the same patterns and behaviour over and over. We think we're doing something different, but we're not. If we put them down sufficiently, they're quite enough that we can start making decisions based on what we really need in life rather than what we think we need.

Then, you know, our attitudes to other people are based on the fact that we're armoured, so we need to be defensive, so why did she say this or he do that? Following the medicine, we can see that it's a softer deal. The edges are not so hard; there are greys in between. There are definitely shades of grey. From someone who was always black-and-white my whole life, there's definitely shades of grey.

This work cannot guarantee the outcomes we may desire, and Fearless's hopes that his wife might be restored to him were not fulfilled.

As problematic as the resulting divorce has been, he continues to draw upon the richness of the personal information with which he has been gifted in the medicine sessions. After the session starts the work, and to our experience, the most fruitful way to embed the insights and epiphanies gained during the session is to take time immediately following the session to allow the material to land in our 'non-medicine' body. This liminal period, when we are slightly under the medicine's influence but increasingly returning to ordinary consciousness, is the ideal time for us to understand and integrate the session material just received. This is especially true if the relaxation is not time-limited and allowed to continue into sleep, the ultimate integrator.

•　•　•

Something enormous in me had suddenly come out or been lifted or released.

Ben W.

This client had been referred by a mutual friend of ours and colleague of his in the financial sector. He was struggling to stay viable for his children after the humbling loss of a robust income following a devastating divorce, and he approached the work sincerely but gingerly. He did not flinch throughout his single session and was able to experience "a depth of understanding...that I had not known I possessed," which "opened me up to myself at some deep level and allowed me to complete a task that had occupied me for many years."

By the age of sixty-two, I had no experience with MDMA. Its street name, ecstasy, led me to believe it was a recreational drug in which I had no interest. I had, at one time, been a regular, long-term, and sometimes heavy user of alcohol, but had quit its use entirely seven years earlier. I was not using any drugs of any kind.

Coming through a difficult breakup, and still struggling with a legacy of childhood violence at the hands of my father many years before, I was told by a friend that perhaps I should explore MDMA in a clinical setting with the help of a longtime practitioner he knew, and under whose guidance he felt he had made great strides in coming to terms with himself.

I made efforts to meet this practitioner to question him extensively on the clinical purity of the medicine, its historical uses, and experiences that others had had in his presence. Duly satisfied with his responses, I decided to embark on a one-time experience.

He prepared me by saying that MDMA would not introduce anything new to my thoughts. It would have no hallucinogenic properties. It would not cause me to think or feel or perceive anything that was not already present in me in some form, at some level. It would induce and facilitate, he said, "a meeting with myself."

I took the MDMA at his suggested dosage, covered my eyes with eyeshades to keep out any light, lay down on a couch in a dimly lit and quiet room, and proceeded to let the drug take hold. About one hour after the first dosage, I took a second, lesser amount.

I cannot detail precisely what happened in sequence, as I was discouraged from taking notes (my wont as a former journalist) or speaking much, but I was aware of becoming settled in my body as if my physical and mental/emotional self was fully awake in three dimensions for the first time. I might have been liquefied or converted to a solid kind of gas in which I was aware of my own occupancy. Nothing felt required by way of movement to become any more comfortable. I was not inclined to sleep, but did not feel so much awake as aware.

It is difficult to characterise extreme levels or depths of awareness, for what is more aware than aware? Suffice it to say that
as time progressed into a second and third hour, I felt myself
both contained and released from all containment into a sensation of my body floating in a sensation of floating. From time
to time, I asked my attendant to write down random thoughts,
which seemed important in that moment, but the core of the
experience was yet to arrive.

I saw myself, or rather my awareness was aware of me, suddenly
in a large lecture hall, the sort of semi-circular and elevated audience arena that many of us encountered in university. Across
the front of the room extended a green chalkboard perhaps six
feet tall and twenty feet across.

Someone or some set of people had been trying to work out
equations of some kind, at different points in time and with
different levels of sophistication suggested by the calculations.
It seemed to me that three or four core problems were being
worked on. Suddenly, I was aware that these were my problems,
that I had been working on them my entire life, and now I could
see, or rather could feel, a unified solution to all of them all at
once. If the calculations on the board represented a search for
answers, the sensation that overcame me was one of a solution
to all these problems simultaneously, and virtually without any
energy or effort. This came in a kind of slow flash, followed by
a sense of quiet contentment. The room or lecture hall that I
was in was in me, and now it was outside me, and so were the
calculations and the solution. Something enormous in me had
suddenly come out or been lifted or released.

My description here may make this experience sound more rational than it was. I was aware of drifting or floating into myself, my thoughts clear and untroubled, and then the image of the lecture hall presented itself, along with every character and function on the chalkboard, all the formulaic and random scribblings. Somehow, the sense of solution emanated from the board, the board within me, the lecture hall outside of me, the "proof" evident in the calculations, and this was mine forever, from that moment, to carry forward with a sense that these problems required no more attention. What relief!

During the hour or two in which the session tailed off, I felt a delicious sense of relaxation and I drifted off to sleep. When I woke, I felt enveloped in a peaceful state. As days passed, I felt something permanently lifted, some level of deep anxiety eased, perhaps forever, and no real impulse to repeat the experience. I would say that without looking for any specific "cure" for any specific "problem," I had found an answer to something that had long been troubling me. I would say that this medicine opened me up to myself at some deep level and allowed me to complete a task that had occupied me for many years.

I was fully awake in three dimensions for the first time.

As I have reflected further on this, I believe that aspects of trauma in my early life, which had interfered with my feelings about myself as well as feelings for others (and on which I had spent many years of talk therapy), were assuaged by this experience. It came to me in the form of mathematical calculations amidst complexity, stationed in a room of higher learning, but from a depth of understanding in me that I had not known I possessed. It was "a meeting with myself" in which deep understanding, long in development, was suddenly revealed.

In this coherent account of his single MDMA session, the client's journalistic skills are evident front and centre. His 'problem' was represented symbolically, and released once it had been understood and owned by him. "As days passed, I felt something permanently lifted, some level of deep anxiety eased, perhaps forever." This is the psyche's normal mechanism-of-action, to decisively release the trauma that it had effectively captured to protect us from its deleterious effects. Once this action occurs, the genie is out of the bottle, and the trauma will not be re-captured, because there is no biological need for the psyche to do so. If elements of the trauma do remain and arise going forward, they are neutered traces that can be managed with further sessions and mindfulness. In this instance, the events were internal to the client and obscure to the attendant in-session, but fully experienced by him and subsequently shared. The post-facto nature of his acceptance of these release events speaks to the medicine's ability to release us from the effects of our traumatic memories, known or forgotten, literally before we know it. Our only role is to show up for ourselves in the first instance by our pivot to approach the work, and then to surrender in-session to the medicine's sweet influence. We release nothing; we are released.

●　●　●

He was a doctor, and so I trusted him.

Alvin P.

From Alvin's considerable experience with the various psychophar-maceutical drugs prescribed to him by psychiatrists for over a decade, post-session he expressed the astonishment many individuals feel when they first experience MDMA. His familiarity with the action of many of the prescription drugs he had been prescribed allowed him, when we spoke at the end of his first medicine session, to reference authoritatively the ability of benzodiazepines (Ativan, Xanax, etc.) to relieve anxiety. He said, "MDMA does for depression what ben-zodiazepines do for anxiety." For a large part of his medicine session, the depression he had felt as a consistent weight throughout his life was simply absent; he experienced himself for the first time without depression. With this encouragement to pursue this medicine work, his path was strewn with the obstacles created by chronic prescription drug use that are contraindicated when working with this medicine. It took a lot of forward planning for him to be clear enough of these suppressive compounds to continue the work.

When I arrived for my first MDMA session with an attendant, it was ten years after a psychiatrist sternly warned me to stay away from ecstasy. The doctor was quizzing me about drug and alcohol use during our first meeting. I was recently out of college. I had come to him for treatment for obsessive compulsive disorder (OCD). I had never taken ecstasy. I had dabbled in other illegal drugs, and I answered honestly, but he only seemed to be concerned about ecstasy. He warned me that it destroyed serotonin receptors and could cause permanent depression. I listened carefully. He was a doctor, and so I trusted him.

I can remember OCD symptoms beginning for me around age ten. My earliest memory of their torment was playing a computer car game and having the sense that I needed to keep playing the game or something bad would happen to my parents. I knew this to be an irrational belief, and so the OCD was ego-dystonic even in its origins, but the anxiety was aggressive, and so I fed it in the same way one scratches an itch that cries louder when it is ignored. I scratched the itch to make the anxiety go away, but the anxiety would not abate, and the condition would expand and feed on itself until it had subsumed me.

As a child, I managed the behaviours, and no one, not even my parents, noticed my inner struggle. Outwardly, I retraced steps, avoided cracks in the sidewalk, agonised over irrelevant details, retied my shoe laces until they frayed and broke, counted incessantly, cracked my thumb knuckles repeatedly, retraced my writing until I made holes in the page (my imperfect handwriting tormented me), and had great difficulty reading, because I was constantly compelled to go backwards to confirm inane details (e.g., the colour of the girl's shirt eight scenes back). Inwardly, I struggled with intrusive thoughts that metastasised and became divorced from the underlying root fear.

I had no language to explain my struggle, even to myself, until I read an article about OCD in the newspaper toward the end of my senior year of high school. I broke down upon reading it and took the article to my parents. Shortly thereafter, my mother arranged for me to see a psychologist. I was leaving soon for college and so only saw the therapist for a handful of meetings. Kind and welcoming, he looked like a mashup of a hippie and a bachelor from the 1970s. I vividly remember him explaining to me that when you push feelings down, they come back up sideways as psychological symptoms, and that in order to resolve the symptoms, you have to fully feel the feelings.

Soon after arriving at college, I went to the school's counselling centre, where I was assigned to a psychiatrist. I don't recall if I knew the difference at that time between a psychologist and a psychiatrist. In the first session, I articulated my symptoms, and the doctor explained to me that I had a biological brain disorder. She recommended that I take Prozac to treat it.

Over the next several years, I went in and out of treatment, going on and off Prozac and trying different antidepressants to treat the OCD, without material affect. Having now become aware of OCD, I worked very hard on my own to suppress the compulsive behaviour. I had success doing that, but the intrusive and obsessive thoughts became increasingly distressful to me. I can remember driving alone in my car, screaming out loud for the intrusive thoughts to stop.

Eventually, I began to see a psychiatrist I would stay with for a number of years. He reiterated that I had a biological brain disorder and told me that I would need to take medication for the rest of my life. Taking psychoactive drugs every day did not sit well with me, particularly when they weren't effectively addressing the problem. I would express my reservations until one session, where the psychiatrist convinced me with some slight exasperation seeping through, that my resistance was an expression of the underlying OCD that needed treatment. The deeper part of me that knew better survived that exchange, but it was silenced and buried for a very long time.

Over the better part of the next ten years, I fought continuously to live a normal life, but it was as if I had two hands tied behind my back. My quality of life and my ability to function oscillated and then deteriorate markedly. Early on, I developed insomnia and was put on sleeping pills. Then, I started to have debilitating anxiety attacks and was put on benzodiazepines. I tried many different antidepressants. When the years passed and nothing seemed to work, it was suggested that I had bipolar disorder II, and I was put on antipsychotics in addition to antidepressants. When I eventually complained that it had become difficult to focus, I was put on a twice daily dose of Adderall.

I was then on five classes of psychiatric drugs simultaneously, all at very high levels. I eventually unravelled and fell into an episode of severe depression that left me largely bedridden for a full year. The head of the psychiatry department at a major hospital tried treating me with oxycodone. A later psychopharmacologist treated me with lithium and suggested a possible Asperger's condition when I described the difficulties I was having functioning. I was hospitalised for depression after the same doctor told me he wasn't sure he still believed in psychopharmacology and took me off my antidepressants without tapering me down. A second psychopharmacologist made the same mistake a year and a half later. A tornado of drug withdrawal symptoms overwhelmed me, and I, again, ended up in the hospital after I swallowed two bottles of pills amidst the confusion.

By the time this period was over, I was ravaged, both psychologically and spiritually. The list of drugs I had been on was four pages long. Nothing worked and everything just kept getting worse for me. By the time the psychiatrists started recommending electroconvulsive therapy (ECT), my faith in them had already been shaken, and, thankfully, I had the strength to refuse it.

It was in this condition that I arrived for my first MDMA treatment session. My first experience was blissful and beautiful and filled with love and ease and grace. It was everything that I had been starved for and had forgotten. It was filled with longing for connection and friendships that had withered. There were no profound psychological or spiritual breakthroughs that would cure me in one session, but my body, mind and soul were bathed in peace for an afternoon. The medicine gave me the hope and relief that I had been longing for, even if just for a few hours.

Over the next two years, I would work with MDMA and with different psychedelic medicines on and off, intensively at first and then a handful of times intermittently. This was a tumultuous and dangerous period for me, during which I felt my sanity was threatened. Stuck between two worlds, I was trying to get off the psychiatric drugs, but the biological model of my condition was still ingrained deeply in my identity. Although the sessions were often very powerful, my symptoms were not improving. A second involuntary hospitalisation after a severe dysphoric episode left me very rattled. I couldn't stay off the psychiatric drugs for more than a few days, and I became increasingly despondent, suffering so intensely that I started to question reality and to believe that my only reason for existing was to suffer.

After a period of time away from the work, a powerful psilocybin session brought to me a realisation that I was not only dependent on psychiatric drugs, but also on psychiatry and its fatalistic worldview. After that session, a deeper part of me emerged, and I was finally able to stay off the drugs for more than a few days. After about a week, I went into a period of intense drug withdrawal that required medical attention. Several days later, I woke up in the middle of the night to an ego death experience. I went back to sleep and then woke up in the morning spontaneously healed. This was a religious experience for me, and I was miraculously well for two full weeks. Unfortunately, the morning after I returned to work, I woke up without energy to get out of bed.

Still determined, I believed I could be suffering from protracted drug withdrawal. I sought out addiction psychiatrists, because I thought they would be sympathetic to my belief that the psychiatric drugs were harmful to me. Instead of helping me detox my system, they nudged me back down the same path I had been trying so hard to get off. I slid back into severe depression, and the next six months would be very painful. In the midst of a dysphoric attack, I swallowed an overdose of sleeping pills. I immediately sought help and was hospitalised for the night. The attending psychiatrist openly mocked me when I said I wasn't taking psychiatric medications, because I thought they were harmful to me. I would be further demoralised when a therapist I had been seeing for a number of years also did not support my thesis.

I became increasingly hopeless and angry and became estranged from my family. Utterly despondent, I moved out of the city to an apartment near the beach. There, I read a memoir by a physician about opiate addiction, and the patients he worked with. I identified fully with the stories of the patients, and the shambles the drugs made of their lives. I was particularly struck by one passage in the book where the internist recounted a psychiatrist telling him that you don't know what a patient's organic psychology is until the patient is off drugs for ninety days.

I stopped taking psychiatric drugs for a second time. This time, it would stick, and I would never see a psychiatrist again. After a period of time, my insomnia lifted, and I slept organically for the first time in a decade. Every morning when I woke up, I marvelled at how I was able to sleep normally again. Organic sleep was truly a miracle for me, and it opened the doors to recovery. My depression quickly lifted. Within a few months, my OCD broke, and I was free of it for the first time since I was a child.

I repaired my relationships with my family. I retrained myself in my field, and I quickly found freelance work and have worked regularly since. As I came upon the close of my first year of recovery, I started to date again. Over the next several years, I continued to rebuild my life. Free of psychiatric drugs, I was able to work directly on the unresolved traumas that had been repressed deep inside of me for decades. Anxiety continued to be a significant issue for me, and as I reached deeper layers of my psyche, shame started to surface as a core issue.

It had been over a year since my last session, when I took MDMA again with an eye toward working on shame. I had no greater expectations than I had for earlier sessions. Shortly after the medicine came on, the origin stories of my psyche began to surface. Volumes of repressed early childhood biographical material broke into my consciousness. All the core material that surfaced in this session would have been unreachable through many lifetimes of traditional therapy.

I did three more MDMA sessions over the next five months, spacing them out by at least one month each time. Each session picked up from the one prior and each alone was far more productive than I had ever imagined a medicine session could be. The first two of the four each surfaced an origin story from very early childhood that dramatically shaped my psyche and explained intimacy issues that plagued me since childhood. The third session surfaced more content related to the first two and helped me to tie everything together.

After the first of these sessions, I was hopeful that all my anxiety and discomfort would disappear fully. This was not the case. In addition to the biographical material, these sessions surfaced deeper and deeper levels of shame, discomfort, tension, numbness, and emotional pain, all of which I experienced in my body. The shame itself felt intensely strange and discordant, like when you hit your funny bone as a child. In addition, these sessions also unearthed layers of anger and a deep-seated and pervasive sense of helplessness, both of which I had to process psychologically.

In the fourth MDMA session of this group, the core belief driving my pain surfaced shortly after the material came on. As I eased into the session, I realised that "something is wrong with me" was the belief that had been driving all my pain for so many years. While I had cognitive awareness that I had deep insecurities for some time, this was a qualitatively different experience. The sense of defectiveness was now coming to me from the source, rather than from an inference made by my adult intellectual mind. I had reached the walled off part of me that was overwhelmed by shame when I was a small child.

While there was no spontaneous deliverance from my pain, now that I had recovered the lost parts of myself, I could soothe them and finally begin to heal my deepest wounds.

The struggle Alvin describes to overcome and reverse the deleterious health effects from a decade of prescription drugs is heroic. As much as outcomes from this work can be decisive, the path to unfold, developmental trauma can be excruciating, taking the individual on twists and turns as the many levels of the trauma are revealed. However, by staying with MDMA work and augmenting it with psilocybin, he was able over some years to bring coherence to his state of being.

A talented and introspective individual, Alvin applied his intelligence to figure out for himself what his individual structures were and identify his false belief that there was 'something wrong' with him. Absent any clarity about what has happened to us, we can only conclude that we, ourselves, are the problem, leaving us vulnerable to believe what we are told by individuals who purport to know, in his case that he had an untreatable 'biological brain disorder.' Respectfully, this is crap; the radical dysfunction Alvin had experienced throughout his life was a product of shame dating back to his first days of life. The Hippocratic Oath to 'Do No Harm' is not only upended by the false diagnosis but compounded by the application of drugs to ameliorate the phantom condition. This doubling-down on wilfully ignorant conclusions by prescribing powerful drugs to treat a nonexistent condition can only result in the chaotic trajectory endured for over a decade of this young man's life.

I felt, for the first time in my life, fully integrated.

Peter G.

One young man had come to the work after an insight that occurred when he was spending time with his daughter following a divorce. His own father had committed suicide when he was eighteen, and he had felt no grief, or anything else, since. One day with his daughter, he was horrified to realise that she understood that he could not feel anything and was compensating for him, and from this moment he knew that he needed to address this terrible lack. This project continues with increasing somatic awareness.

Peter, the individual whose testimony follows and who has also worked with us, has had no access to his feelings for his entire life, and the following account of his work in-session and in-life is noteworthy. Following both medicine sessions and his committed meditation practice, he is able to bring pin-point focus to the task of evoking feeling. He once teared up during a conversation and remarked there and then how this occurrence gave him joy; he could feel.

I have not had the same experience with emotions that everyone else seems to have. I don't feel emotions in the way that everyone else does. Looking back, I realise that's been the case with me from a very young age, perhaps since infancy. That clearly manifested in my behaviour. There are less extremes of behaviour.

In a way, I was vaguely aware that the world, as I experienced it, was black-and-white, and that the colour and texture, emotional valence that everyone else was attuned to, I was not; there was a richness of experience to which I had no exposure. I had an intuition that not only was my life experience poorer as a result, but my behaviour might not be as good as it would be were I also able to feel emotion. I didn't feel as close to my immediate family members as I otherwise would have. Perhaps even negative emotions, had I felt them, would have been better to have than the general sense of not having feelings.

The first time that I experienced MDMA was a complete revelation. It wasn't just that under the medicine I was feeling things stronger than usual. Rather, it was that I was feeling feelings to begin with! I felt great ecstatic joy and overwhelming love for my own children, which I had never felt. Not even a minuscule amount of this emotion for my children had I been consciously aware of before, or experienced even a taste of before. It was an experience of complete joy and ecstasy and revelation and a feeling of connection and attunement between mind and body. Under the medicine, my body was dancing to music, and my mind was hearing the same music as my body and feeling integrated with it. I felt, for the first time in my life, fully integrated. I didn't even know before that experience that until then I'd been unintegrated. I just had no notion of my body at all. I mean, I felt physical sensation, but I had no sense that my body was an alive entity that my mind was fused with as opposed to being simply an organic appendage and tool of my mind.

I returned home as the medicine started wearing off. For the rest of the evening, in my interactions with my wife and my kids, I felt extremely present, and I felt a unity with them that I'd never felt before, that we were an integrated family, one whole cohesive unit. I experienced enjoying spending time with them and just being with them and being involved in the activities that they wanted to be involved in and just enjoying the experience of being with my family members such that I'd never felt even one iota of before. When the medicine wore off, I no longer felt like that. I no longer behaved like that with my wife and kids. I had a memory of that, of course, and I knew that's how I wanted to be. That was the way I briefly was under the medicine, and that was the way I should be, and that was the way I was entitled to be, and my family deserved me to be.

I have a strong meditation practice. When I was on the medicine, I discovered that the feeling, the emotion of joy, was strongest in certain parts of my chest and certain parts of my breath. Particularly at the end of my in-breath it was strongest, and also very strong at the end of the out-breath. I also found that the sensation of joy was extremely strong at the edges of my mouth when I was smiling. I found in the succeeding few days, when I was meditating, that if I forced a smile and aimed my attention in the corners of my mouth, I was able, when I was very, very quiet in meditation, to sense a very, very, very faint tingling of joy—that same joy that I only ever experienced on the medicine a few days before and perhaps ever so faintly on just two other occasions in my adult life.

Over a period of weeks, by aiming and sustaining at the corners of my mouth, I was able to grow that tingling sensation of joy, just like kindling a fire and from a spark, I was able to sustain a very, very small fire. The sensation grew bigger, I could hold it, just like kindling a fire from a spark. I kindled that spark and sustained it into a very, very small fire. And then I found I was able to somehow drop that sensation from the corners of my mouth into my chest, and so feel that sensation of joy in my chest. And that was the first time in my life, other than that time a week or two earlier when I'd been on the medicine, that I had experienced a sensation of joy in my body. An incredible experience.

Unfortunately, I have been able to do that only in deep meditation and not yet off of the cushion. But in other work, I'm hoping to bring that into my everyday life.

Over the years, I've seen many different therapists from different schools of therapy and obviously thought about my absence of emotion, and I've had various theories about why this deficiency arose in me in the first place in my young childhood or infancy. It was truly remarkable to me that I could suddenly have access, and such powerful access, to something I'd been missing my whole life in just one sitting, in one morning and afternoon. I guess, for me, a large part of the solution is being able to experience it, to have set foot in the promised land, to have had this experience that I've heard and read and seen others experience all the time made tangible for me. It makes it easier for me to set my sights and chart my course to arrive there eventually, I hope, without needing medicine.

I would say my body had been in a deep sleep, if not a coma, for decades, and what the medicine did was to awaken me from that coma for several hours and then put me back to sleep, but not in as deep a sleep as I had been before. And with awakening is a consciousness that a permanent awakening may be possible. Over the succeeding months, through meditation and through more medicine, my body has started to wake up. My body feels only fully awake when I'm on medicine, but even when I'm not on medicine, other than feeling in a coma, it just feels very tired. But it definitely seems that the body is eventually on a path to fuller awakening, even without medicine.

This work is, itself, meditation, and Peter's skillful co-mingling the feelings he had enjoyed under the medicine within his meditations, as well as the focus he brings to bear on the tiniest sensations, is remarkable. It is also fruitful and speaks clearly to the interrelatedness of medicine work and meditation and demonstrates how this complimentary relationship may be used to clarify and further explore the meaning of content revealed in-session.

It also underscores the proposal that contemplatives are the natural fit for supervision of work with MDMA that necessitates quiet, minute-to-minute attendance over the many hours of the session.

Peter continues the work with his customary diligence. During one session, he asked, "Where is my mother's love?" A few minutes later he asked, "Is there love at all?" It is impossible and even redundant to try to fathom how a child could not feel any love at all, but this dreadful void had determined his life. In one meditation session, he experienced himself as a black-and-white picture frame that lacked its image of colourful flesh and blood that comprise the body. Blessedly, nothing is lost, it is just lost to us. For Peter to experience feelings of love and joy under the medicine affirmed his own organic ability to feel, and he understood that his inability to experience feelings in life was in no way a deficit in himself but an artefact of some unknown

deficit in his upbringing. This understanding has led to his quiet,
fierce and righteous endeavour to carry the medicine work forward
and to address his condition with meditation that is revealing to
him, little by little, the actual feeling of love from which he has been
so cruelly absented his whole life.

• • •

I've wanted to get to this place forever.

Wylie M.

Wylie's description of his single session is a simple, eloquent statement of the healing power of MDMA. His testimony conveys the internal feeling of being under the influence of this medicine exquisitely. His sincerity in approaching the work, his 'set,' was rewarded with a recalibration of his psychic structure that has resulted, after many years of effort in other realms, in coherence of mind and body.

The first words out of my mouth while working with the powerful healing medicine, MDMA, were, "I've wanted to get to this place forever." This 'place' I had been searching for is an undeniable feeling of self-love and gratitude. These feelings materialised and swept over my body within thirty minutes of ingestion. It felt familiar, feelings that had always been there but always unfelt, inhabiting my body, ready to show me the beautiful power of acceptance, trust, and love.

That inherent state of being, my natural self, had been repressed for three decades underneath layers of unresolved traumas, and blanketed by pesky distractions, working hard to assure that I not leave a comfortable state of avoidance. I believe this immediate awareness is unequivocal evidence of the power of MDMA and its capacity to facilitate a remarkable transformation. Eureka!

Like many others, I too, exhausted countless attempts to heal through psychotherapy, prescription drugs, acupuncture, acupressure, diet, exercise, meditation, to name a few. While I commend my efforts and have certainly made positive changes as a result, still I felt like I was not living an abundant life. The problem is that these methods mainly focus on my symptoms—depression, negativity, avoidance, fear, impulsive behaviour, and distractions. I was interested in exploring the source, but only from an intellectual context, not from a physical whole body perspective.

After spinning wheels for far too long, I began to shift my focus and understand the importance and intelligence of the subtle body. What I learned is that if you listen carefully, the body will tell you exactly what it needs. I also learned that certain substances, if taken in the right set and setting with mindful intentions, can act as a portal to connecting to feelings in the body in a more profound way. I was attracted to MDMA because of its gentle nature. I began researching more and learned about MDMA's pure intentions, which does not include raves, glow sticks, and electronic music. Its real intention is to teach acceptance, love, and trust. It's a powerful enabler of the unadulterated true self, free of societal conditioning.

My experience with MDMA did not disappoint my expectations.

In fact, it far exceeded what I thought was possible. The experience was so caring, reassuring, and beautiful. It gently guided me through a self-explorative landscape by lowering my anxiety and heightening my awareness. I found that basic goodness exists deep inside myself, as well as in all beings. It connected me to my peers, subordinates, friends, and family by showing me that we are all connected. It awakened a deep sense of empathy and forgiveness that is infinite and enduring. I gained new insights into past experiences, which allowed me to feel more forgiveness and to become free of shame. It felt safe, loving, and supportive to my healing process; lasting healing that I hold with me today.

Moving forward, I understand that the work does not end with the culmination of the non-ordinary state. The real work begins the next day, week and months, integrating what I have learned into my life. I am in the process of rebuilding from a new foundation, a new foundation that is free from the restrictions of shame and self-hatred, along with many other symptoms that kept me distracted and unable to fully experience life. I have a greater capacity to love myself and all beings. With this greater capacity, I am uncovering other areas of my life that I would like to work on and evolve. I feel more in control. I accept suffering. A different kind of suffering; a voluntary suffering that is necessary for long-term growth.

Wylie is continuing the healing trajectory begun with MDMA, gratefully accepting the ongoing task of integration from 'a new foundation.' He found that place of 'acceptance, trust, and love' within him that he had wanted to get to forever, a considerable achievement precipitated through the blessing of the medicine. In truth, this feeling 'of self-love and gratitude' is also who we are, but through God-knows-what occurrences in our early life has become unreachable to us. Since his session, Wylie has moved from working in the real estate industry that was meaningless to him and has found work with organisations promoting socially useful agendas that he finds both meaningful and rewarding.

CHAPTER SIX

Trust, Surrender, Receive

———

*"To be wholesome we must remain truthful to
our vulnerable complexity. In order to keep
our balance we need to keep the interior and
exterior, visible and invisible, known and
unknown, temporal and eternal, together. No
one else can undertake this task for you. You are
the one and only threshold of an inner world."*

JOHN O'DONOHUE, ANAM CARA

The client's ability first to trust, second to surrender, and third to receive are essential to the successful outcomes of their therapeutic work with MDMA. The three stages overlap, but they are distinct.

TRUST

"Basic trust is a non-conceptual confidence in the goodness of the universe, an unquestioned implicit trust that there is something about the universe and human nature and life that is inherently and fundamentally good, loving and wishing us the best. This innate and unformulated trust in life and reality manifests as a willingness to take that plunge into the abyss." A. H. Almaas

Trust is a basic human need. Trust is foundational in any interaction—with a friend, a store clerk, or other drivers on the highway. In an MDMA session, nothing can proceed without a deep mutual trust between the client and the attendant who will be sitting with them for six or more hours. That trust between them must be carefully cultivated by both parties. The client, particularly, must trust the attendant, the situation, the room, the process, the medicine, and the whole endeavour. In the absence of complete trust, no medicine session can be undertaken.

In his book *Facets of Unity*, the spiritual teacher A.H. Almaas talks about the fundamental need for trust. He suggests, without trust, we have lost a fundamental aspect of our being that will impact our development going forward. The need goes back to the very beginning of our lives; if we cannot trust our mothers to hold us and love us, our capacity to trust others throughout our lives is compromised. Almaas calls this "basic trust" and says that most of us have some of it and some of us have a lot of it. Some of us, however, have very little trust, precisely because it's been violated.

Consider, from your position as an adult, a young child who experiences violence at the hands of a caretaker. If a fearful event occurs, we are changed. It is not an act of will but of the body's instantaneous response to the circumstance, and our attention becomes focused on the threat, until we discern that it has passed. Survival instinct. Now, if such a fear-producing threat or threats occurred when we were a youngster, and that fear is captured by the psyche's action to protect us (per Unexperienced Experience), then we live from a foundation of fear. Every thought, word, and deed is conditioned by fear, and fear-based decisions are, in every case, the worst decisions. A child conditioned by fear is at a dreadful disadvantage in their development and throughout their lives. This is how the imprint of trauma, unbeknownst to us, can affect us in ways that determine our behaviour.

Such individuals may never have complete trust again; they have lost their innocence far too early in their development. This loss can precipitate an existential crisis, because the person can no longer experience him- or herself as a discrete entity. They know they are not inviolable, for they have been violated. If it can happen once, it can happen again, and they live with this ever-present fear as a condition every single day of their life.

We see this frequently in our clients. Quite often, they enter the work feeling like they can't trust anything. Trust has become threat. If they have been abused by a parent, for instance, the protective nurturing trust they should have developed simply does not exist. It can be a huge piece of their work just to reach this place of understanding, so they can trust in the medicine, the process, the place, the setting, and the people involved.

On the other hand, people usually come to us after a period of intense reckoning with their situation and consideration of this possible solution. They've heard about the healing potential of MDMA from a friend, a client, or a colleague, and already have a sense that it could be a worthwhile endeavour. Their trust is already building when they contact us the first time. Then, when they understand they will be looked after for the duration of the sessions, there's no pressure on them to 'do' anything, and nobody is going to do anything to them, they can trust a little more.

Our clients go into their sessions with a firm understanding of the process and of potential outcomes. They are highly motivated, because it has simply become so difficult to live with their treatment-resistant condition. The ways they have been dealing with it have all been unsuccessful. Now, with trust in the work itself, in the attendant and the location, they are prepared to expose themselves to the medicine.

SURRENDER

"If you are able to surrender, then you are willing to be. You are willing to not try to change things, to not manipulate them, to not push and pull at them."

A. H. ALMAAS

The trust that is established in our consultations is reinforced on the session day, and up until the moment when they take the first dose, clients are free to bail if they have any doubts or fears at all. In our experience, this has never occurred. Trust is the platform necessary for the client to enter the next stage of the work, their fullest surrender to the experience of the medicine. It is normal to feel a little anxious. After all, we will be going somewhere unfamiliar; who would not be a bit nervous? If necessary, we reassure them, again, of the comforting setting and our constant presence, and we encourage them to relax and to understand they do not have to do anything. The most productive strategy is for them to simply allow the MDMA to approach them, avoid resisting as much as they can, and let the medicine do the work. As Carl Jung has said, "What you resist, persists."

Relaxation sets in as the medicine gently takes effect and grows more pronounced over some time, becoming "full-on" usually around an hour or so. Soon enough, the client moves beyond relaxation to total surrender. They quickly discover that not only is it not a scary place, they may feel better than they have ever felt in their lives.

Our society delivers many messages about surrender, few of them positive. We are told to never surrender, never give up the fight. In this instance, though, we need to surrender our everyday selves to a larger, expanded self that is more knowing and contains information about the trauma from which we have been separated. Surrender allows us to open to the information that has been captured, and to allow those caught and held memories to become part of our somatic and cognitive consciousness for the first time.

A quotation from Aldous Huxley, "The willingness to be completely implicated," captures the readiness to surrender. It is the attitude of, "Okay, if I am going to do this, let me really do it. Let me do this surrendering thing and see what happens." You need to be open to everything you might discover without fear or favour; good, bad, or ugly.

In the medicine session, the client experiences themselves as loving, loved, and lovable. Just the fact that they can relax can represent significant progress for many traumatised people, but with MDMA they not only relax, they soon feel a warm and blissful sense of ease.

There can be bumps in the road; it is not always a smooth transition from stress to surrender. As the medicine slowly begins to take effect, the newness of it all may bring up a panic response for some clients, with fear, heart palpitations, and sweating. This is very rare and is always temporary, lasting only a few minutes. In such cases, the attendant's role is to reassure them and help them through it, perhaps offering a hand to hold or suggesting some breathing to bring equilibrium back to the body.

What we ask clients to do, essentially, is to "relax into the anxiety." One client, who verbalised his tremendous anxiety in the session, was encouraged to do this and gave his attendant a look he will never forget: "What? Are you kidding me?" It was a pivotal moment for him. He now appreciates that surrender is exactly what is needed to revisit and allow release of our traumas.

Some elements of the attendant's strategy deliberately encourage the state of surrender, particularly the use of eyeshades. Donning the eyeshades and blocking out the external world enhances our focus on the internal world and signals the movement from trust to surrender. When the session starts, we offer a little orange juice with which to take the medicine (vitamin C helps cross the blood-brain barrier). We suggest the client take the medicine, put on the eyeshades, and lie down all in one movement. The next forty-five minutes to an hour are the most important for the client as the medicine approaches and establishes the non-ordinary state of consciousness. Once it is established, the client may express surprise and delight. They have a real incentive to stay with it as the condition is so interesting, to say the least. Taking the medicine and staying with it signifies their determination to maintain the focus on their inner condition for the rest of the day. The attendant stays with the client in stillness, and slowly but surely the medicine begins to open them to enable a meeting with themselves.

While the panic attacks mentioned earlier are very rare, some mild anxiety may occur as we wait for the medicine to take effect, and as attendants we encourage the client to focus on the breath, the inhale and the exhale, and to use this like a mantra; "I am breathing." Thich Nhat Hanh suggests on the in-breath to say, "I have arrived," and on the out-breath to say, "I am home."

Most people simply enjoy the chance to have nothing to do and can relax. After about thirty or forty minutes, their breathing may come in big sighs, becoming fuller. They might shift onto their side, or pull their knees up to their waists, or simply lie still.

As attendants, we are sometimes asked if it is not boring for us to sit there, doing nothing, while the client lies motionless on the couch. On the contrary, enabling the healing potential of MDMA is a privilege, as is being able to give someone the opportunity to spend quality time in non-ordinary consciousness. We understand from attendants who have been present for our own work with the medicine that this is best achieved when we take ourselves out of the picture to give the client the clear, uncluttered space they need.

RECEIVE

"The third step is to allow things to develop spontaneously and naturally in the way they want to develop, without trying to channel them in ways that you think they should go."

A. H. ALMAAS

Following their trust and surrender, the client needs to be ready and willing to receive whatever is revealed during the process. We are an acquisitive species and live in a "gimme-gimme" world, so we might think we want to receive whatever emerges. In working with trauma, however, we might get the very material we have been unconsciously protecting ourselves from all our lives. How do you gracefully and productively receive such a gift?

As the Rolling Stones have pointed out, "You can't always get what you want, but if you just might try, you just might find, you get what you need." The guiding principle is to receive without fear or favour. To take a neutral stance, regardless of what memories arise, and give our discernment to the whole organism. That includes body, mind, and spirit. This enables it to deliver the secrets that it has held beyond the reach of our conscious mind. We encourage clients to let whatever comes up just come up; they must trust that the organism has chosen it for a reason, and thus, it is likely to be the most urgent thing we need to address. At a certain point, clients may find it difficult to maintain such equanimity. They might think, "Oh, God, I remember this. It was horrible," but we suggest they hold themselves open for this memory, as terrible as it may be. It is information that is important to them. When we allow these memories to re-emerge, and stay with them for several minutes or even hours, the psyche finally gets a chance to realise that the time of the trauma has passed, and it is safe to release the memories that it had originally captured.

In work with MDMA, the body does the processing. When we talk, we are still in ordinary consciousness and the brain, our cognitive function, is dominant. With the medicine, you are still thinking, but your cognition is no longer in charge. The relationship between your mind and your emotions has been upended, and feelings dominate thinking. The cognitive self is now in a secondary position, subservient to the emotional self that is leading the way. Our habits of thought become exposed to this field of greater informational coherence.

On a practical level, surrendering during an MDMA session means agreeing to stay within the process, even if difficult memories come up. Especially if difficult memories come up, as a matter of fact. Living through those memories is a necessary part of the healing trajectory. It is also a moment when we may realise the impossibility of managing such transitions by ourselves. In truth, we cannot undertake this non-ordinary consciousness work alone, which is why we sit with our clients in the way that we have enjoyed—quietly, respecting the medicine.

We are there to help them receive everything coming their way. If they panic a little, take off their eyeshades and become agitated, we might coax them back to the couch, suggest the eyeshades again, and encourage them to recline and relax. We might encourage them to stay with their discomfort, understanding that the session is time-limited and that we will be with them the whole time. The available presence of a dedicated attendant is essential for them to stay open to receiving anything that comes up. We cannot do this work alone.

TYPES OF TRAUMA

"Perhaps all our dragons are princesses that are just waiting to see us, once, beautiful and brave. Perhaps everything is, in its deepest being, something helpless that wants help from us."

RAINER M. RILKE.

MDMA can be an extremely effective treatment for many traumas, but differences in outcomes may depend upon the type of trauma involved; the ease of release depends on the timing and extremity of the traumatic event or events. Broadly speaking, there are two ways that trauma can be received by the body; from a shock to the system in adulthood, and from developmental trauma during childhood.

SHOCK TRAUMA

Perhaps, when we think of trauma, we think of discrete events like kidnappings, car accidents, rapes, and military battles experienced by adults. Such discrete events, occurring with sudden and terrible ferocity, are called shock trauma. People who endure these terrifying moments tend to be able to remember the facts of the events. Sgt. K. was victim to an IED explosion in Iraq that killed his friends. He was in terrible pain and developed PTSD symptoms from the trauma, but he could still remember the details.

Joining the military was, for him, an act of adult volition; he felt drawn to military service and, as an adult and knowing full-well the risks, he signed up. Twice. During his tours, he was surrounded by his buddies and senior officers as they lived hyper-vigilant under the constant threat of death. So, the memory of the IED explosion, however fractured and incomplete, occurred within a framework of knowing who he was, where he was, what he was doing at the time of the event, and why. When the full emotional horror of what occurred is experienced in the medicine session, the known details support the emerging emotional memory. He reaffirms he was in Helmand Province; there was incoming from Hill 105; the Humvee was an unreinforced piece of shit, etc. This information has kept the experience front and centre in his conscious memory since it happened, and enables the emotional memory to have coherence when it emerges during the session. This allows for a full embrace of the memory, and the psyche's release.

When the details of the traumatic event are known and available to us consciously, MDMA has an easier task of releasing the event. The memories feel coherent to the person experiencing them through the medicine; their feeling of the event comports with their conscious memory of the event. Sometimes the trauma can be released in a single session. Several client testimonies describe this phenomenon.

To our view, this may bode well for the veterans who are suffering from PTSD as the result of their experiences in the theatre of war.

It has been observed that the release outcomes from working with people dealing with shock trauma are clearer and more decisive than for people who suffer from developmental trauma.

DEVELOPMENTAL TRAUMA

Early childhood sexual abuse, physical abuse, or severe neglect throughout childhood fall under the heading of developmental trauma. A child who lives every day under extreme and even frightening conditions, with little or no solace from a parent or caregiver, has no choice but to suppress the fearfulness of their environment and events. A chaotic home life may be normative for them, and that is reflected in their imbalance of their own emotional behaviour. Young children have no agency to ameliorate their own internal traumatic conditions. They can only suck it up and move on as best they can, so the trauma gets deeply buried.

Developmental traumas are more difficult to release, not only because they are cognitively unknown; they are literally embedded in the body. In the case of abuse events, the adult body has grown around the five-year-old's body, and the individual develops in such a way that they are never able to experience themselves free of fear. Similarly, in the case of daily, ongoing, and systemic neglect, the child may have not known any other reality than living in trauma. Their reality may contain both neglect and abuse, compounding the trauma they carry. They come to believe that the problem is themselves, and because trauma is their baseline, they have no way of knowing and understanding the problem was created *by* the trauma.

Sometimes, developmental traumas occur before we even have language to describe them.

Releasing deeply held developmental trauma can be extremely complex, and may require extended work. The work of Bruce Perry, M.D. with severely traumatised children bears witness to the subtlety, patience and delicacy required to ameliorate early traumas.

Some client testimonies reflect this; many have found significant release with MDMA, but developmental trauma can be resistant to full release, and traces may remain embedded, requiring further work.

COMPLEX TRAUMA

Trauma diagnosis seldom fits neatly into one of the two categories above; it is more complex than "either-or" and can be a "both-and" situation. Developmental trauma, for instance, might be further exacerbated by instances of shock trauma. It is not uncommon for clients to present with one type of problem, but discover additional layers over time. The destabilising effects of early developmental trauma may not only make people more vulnerable to shock trauma later, but they can also cause victims to unconsciously "invite" trauma into their lives.

One woman came to the work to address intimations of an incident or incidents of sexual abuse when she was around five years old and brought a snapshot of herself at that age to the session. What emerged, however, was an incident of being sexually violated from having been given a date-rape drug as a young woman. This was a shock trauma event.

Why didn't she recognise what was going on? She came to understand that the earlier sexual abuse had taken away her ability to discern predatory behaviour at all. As a result, she was not able to recognise a predator; he seemed familiar. Shock trauma and developmental trauma can interact, back and forth, reinforcing confusion in the victim.

ONTOLOGICAL SHOCK

"We need to legitimise experience itself."

JOHN E. MACK, M.D.

Dr. John E. Mack, the late Harvard professor of psychiatry and Pulitzer Prize-winning author, focused his professional attention throughout his life toward severely traumatised people who had experienced what he came to understand was "ontological shock." Ontological means "relating to being or existence." Ontological shock is a wound so deep it infuses every layer of our being and colours the very sense of our existence; these victims may experience everything in their environment as a threat to their integrity. A wall is a threat. A person is a threat. People who have been traumatised in early childhood often find themselves in this condition of being unable to truly trust anything or anybody, and shock trauma can result in the same outcome instantaneously. Ontological shock is an extreme and unnatural condition, a cloud of doubt and fear suffusing every aspect of the individual's life resulting in an extremely limited state of being.

Ontological shock can result from both developmental and shock trauma and precipitates an existential crisis in the individual, resulting in doubt, fear, and uncertainty. Who am I if I am constantly being punished and told I am wrong? Who am I if my own body can be violated? Dr. Mack advocated passionately for legitimising the victim's experience, no matter how horrible or fantastic or improbable it may seem to an outsider. It is their experience, and who are we to judge?

Dr. Mack worked with deeply disturbed people who had suffered terribly, something quite beyond their normal ability to integrate, leading to their dysfunctional lives; suicidal teenagers, alcoholics, addicts, and abductees. This open-hearted approach of taking the accounts the latter presented seriously—believing them—met with considerable resistance from some quarters; colleagues doubted the memories associated with their abduction experiences were entirely true. That was beside the point, Mack insisted, and inimical to good clinical practice. To deny someone's experience is to disrespect them, and is also fundamentally irrelevant to any course of action that could lead to healing. Legitimising of every aspect of the client's condition at presentation is crucial to the individual's subsequent ability to allow meaningful experiences that may be beyond their consciousness to emerge in the medicine session.

THE MEANING OF MEMORIES

Clients are frequently surprised by the memories they receive in their MDMA sessions. One woman, whose testimony in her own words appears in this book, realised that her own behaviour was not normal when compared with her teenage peers, and she had worked on her feelings of confusion for over ten years before exposing herself to MDMA therapy. During her session, a series of events that she could never have imagined was illuminated. The client was horrified, but her experience under the medicine was clear, authentic, and importantly, made sense of her behaviours. Getting the whole story was very freeing. She had known she was different and troubled all her life, but she had no explanation for her bizarre behaviours. Now, she knows, and importantly knows that this was not her doing. She has forgiven everybody involved and moved on with her life.

All memories have meaning; without memories, we cannot learn. In the case of captured traumatic memories, we may feel or act out something compulsively without any knowledge of why we are doing so. Our knowledge base tells us one thing, our behaviour another, and this split between one part of ourselves and the other can destabilise our sense of who we are. Further, we cannot learn much of anything, because we do not know the facts of the matter; we are condemned to flounder in a dark cloud of unknowing.

The issue of recovered memories may come up in the client's initial consultation. We reference our non-interventionist approach and ensure him or her that whatever may come up in the medicine session does so only from within him- or herself. This is critically important for the client to understand. We are clear that whatever is revealed during the medicine session, they have often carried all their lives and have brought it with them into the session room.

The attendants, the room, and the whole environment is completely neutral and clean, with no outside suggestions or influences of any kind. We treat every memory that emerges in this work as a true memory of a real event that occurred in the past, an event or events that led to the individual's dysfunction and brought them to work with MDMA. This posture is supported by the fact that in every case where a client has recovered memories of abuse, that knowledge enables the psyche to release. Our role is to maintain a necessary distance and offer support; nothing more. Whatever is shared from the client to the attendant is in that direction alone. The attendant offers nothing, no suggested scenarios or anything else whatsoever that could influence the content of a client's experience.

I was starting to realise what it means to be happy.

Parco Smith

This thoughtful individual references the medicine work and meditation quite interchangeably. His sessions were punctuated throughout with expressions of surprise he expressed conversationally, with remarks marking his progress such as, "I am with my father." He was fully and continuously aware of what was occurring within this meeting with himself, while simultaneously maintaining conscious contact with his attendant. We can enhance the process by maintaining and accepting this dual awareness that greatly assists the psyche to determine that whatever is being revealed within us, we are now in this present moment safe, enabling release.

It had been eighteen years since my first experience with the medicine, when I decided to try it again for different reasons. When I was a teenager living in California, I had done the work probably four or five times and had fond memories; I had attributed a deep personality change within me to my experience at that time, but had still categorised it as belonging to the past, a path to self-discovery and growth taken as a teenager.

I started attending psychotherapy talk therapy sessions to explore a general discontent with my work, personal romantic life, and the relationship with my parents. From the outside, both my work situation (I'd been the director of an art studio for ten years) and my home life (I'd been in a relationship for fifteen years) seemed to indicate that I was happy and fulfilled. I was persistently overwhelmed by a general discontent that I couldn't shake off and a feeling that there was not much I could do about it. I did not know where to start to make the necessary changes.

Besides psychotherapy, I was learning to meditate. In talk therapy, I felt that I wasn't making enough progress, because we discussed topics intellectually rather than allowing actual feelings. I was more in my head, analysing and rationalising, and the feelings weren't quite accessible. I was also beginning to acknowledge the traumatic impact of a dark and abusive upbringing as well as two violent events that occurred later in life. One was an armed robbery, in which I was held hostage without means of escape, and the other was when I witnessed the September 11th terrorist attacks from downtown New York City.

Now, through a dear friend, the opportunity presented itself to re-experience the medicine in an introspective setting with the presence of an attendant. I was excited but at the same time anxious about what the session would be like. The anxiety emerged from various thoughts.

First, I felt guilty that I was requesting a day off from work for what in my mind still seemed like something self-centred.

Second, I had concerns about the effect of the medicine on my heart rhythm, and whether I could handle it. This was a symptom of what I self-diagnosed as my light hypochondriacal tendency.

Third, although some friends who I had informed about what I intended to do were supportive, others were highly sceptical and helped create the perception that I was about to jump into the vast unknown.

On the day of the session, I sat on the prepared couch with a blanket, pillow, and blindfold. On the coffee table were two small ceramic dishes. I swallowed the first pill, while the attendant started the music that would accompany the journey for the next five hours.

I put on my blindfold and lay back on the couch, eagerly awaiting the feeling of the medicine as I had remembered it from my teenage years. I was constantly asking myself if this was it, if it had started to take effect. Around twenty minutes in, I felt the first rushing wave flowing through my body. This was it. Unmistakably, I was feeling the effects of the medicine. I started breathing as I do while meditating or during yoga, taking deep breaths into my belly. I was letting the medicine do its work and trying not to focus on whether my heart was beating too fast or not. Initially, I had to go to the bathroom multiple times; the medicine is a diuretic, and I was making sure to drink enough water.

When I noticed that Spanish guitar music was playing, I immediately had a strong dislike for it, because it reminded me of my father. I almost asked for the music to be changed, but decided to work through what I was experiencing as a very un-pleasurable situation. Why didn't I want to listen to that song? Why didn't I want to be reminded of my father?

It was obvious why.

After around ninety minutes, the attendant suggested the possibility of taking the next dose. I had some apprehension, because the first dose felt quite strong, but he said to take my time and do it only if and when I felt like it.

When I felt ready, I took the second dose and relaxed. An encompassing feeling of the universe ebbing and pulsating took over. Now, I was in a place so comfortable, so relaxed, simply breathing. Enjoying each breath, enjoying my hands touching my arms, caressing myself. What was happening was so beautiful, and the very fact that I could admit that it was beautiful was groundbreaking. I had always been so scared to allow any emotions, but now, I was realising that it was okay to feel and to admit I had feelings. And guess what? I acknowledged to myself that it felt great to be me. Why had I never felt like this before? I had no idea; I had spent my life walking around feeling so inferior, so tense, so anxious.

Soon enough, however, the main reason this had been the case became apparent. I had incorporated a general social construct of being an outsider and not being normal, because of my sexuality and my cultural heritage. After this realisation, I felt as if I was looking from the outside toward myself, as well as from within myself. And suddenly all the structures and ideas that I had incorporated subliminally about who I was became apparent. The origin of these ideas I identified as being society and parents, but it was my mind that had implemented them. And there was no reason to, because they were superficial, materialistic, and ephemeral. They did not concern the true reality of Being. What it means to be a human being, pure, faultless, and full of love. Suddenly, I recognised that love is the true connection between human beings and that all divisive thoughts come from controlling external structures. I could see that ideas, like the idea of "the American Dream," are controlling; I called it the ultimate colonisation of the mind. I could see geopolitical boundaries and structures of mind-control that delineate and divide human against human.

The idea of money and power became clear; how it is so divisive and the source of so many people feeling inferior about themselves. I was one of them. But now, I saw through it and was able to release its power over me.

I was able to realise that I don't need to look at career, money, or education level to feel as if I am a complete human being worth something. I was already complete. Everything else is great to engage in, but it is not the ultimate reality. We do not need to have external factors dictate how we feel about ourselves. And if some things are beyond our reach financially, it is okay. We will be fine, because what matters is already inside of us, not the external objectives inculcated into us since childhood by our parents and our culture.

I was starting to realise what it means to be happy. True happiness, you only achieve from within. No one will give you that. Acceptance comes from within. These ideas sound like clichés, and I knew them intellectually, but what this medicine was doing was making me feel that I was truly happy with myself, from within, and that I could be like that every day, because the only cause for me not feeling complete would be an external cause, something learned, artificial, and temporary.

A strong lightning storm began a few hours into the experience, and I noticed the thunder. I felt as if I was floating in the atmosphere within the clouds and that the thunder and lightning were all around me; I was part of it. Nature. It was all the same. Then, I had the vision of me being a moss and my father a rock. I realised that the moss can grow however it wants and that it doesn't choose the rock, but it can still grow on top. It doesn't need much from the rock, and it can exist with it in peace. I was coming to terms with my father; what he had done to me as a child could now be forgiven, and my need for love from him was no longer a matter of my survival or of me feeling complete. I could now see myself reestablishing a bond and a relationship with my father based not on anger but on love.

I was also working on my creativity and noticing the music, how free it seemed. It was all about sound and space. I acknowledged that I had a musical block. I had adopted aesthetic notions or ideals that were restraining me from truly expressing myself. I was so worried about what other people would think. This is how I was carrying myself in life as well, and now I could see that it was all in my mind; I was creating the self-limiting scenario. I was the critic, so self-critical in fact that I was not allowing myself to create or to do anything to feel whole.

I did think about my childhood and the traumatic life events that had happened, but they didn't seem to be bothersome. I was realising that they had been traumatic, yes, and that I had been pretending they were normal and ordinary.

I felt as if I had gained more insight than from five years in talk therapy. The important aspect wasn't that I was thinking of all these ideas, but that I was feeling them. I was feeling complete. I felt that I was okay and now I could begin to heal and grow into my real self. All my interests and aspirations can now flourish, because the self-limiting critic inside me has lost its power.

I describe this session as meditation in a pill. I now felt that I truly understood how to meditate properly; watching feelings and thoughts come and go while remaining present, not pushing them away, but acknowledging them.

It is now two years since this first session, and I feel so vastly improved. I have developed my spiritual beliefs. I have a general feeling that I can change things in my life that are not working, more confidence to address difficult emotions and subjects. I have also improved the way that I relate to friends, family, and strangers, always trying to relate with a more compassionate and empathic perspective. I meditate regularly and life generally doesn't seem as overwhelming as it did before my session, and at the same time, I have greater access to my feelings.

We can see the essential role that meditation can play in integrating the insights from this work demonstrated in Parco's testimony, and for sure all attendants are committed contemplatives. Whatever has been caught and held within us, internalised often for many years, is going to need some consideration of time, some serious patience to resolve. Even when release is instantaneous, feelings resulting from the release may occur also requiring our attention, and the open space offered in meditation is the ideal forum within which they may arise and be processed.

● ● ●

To live in such anguish was not an option.

S. S.

The crippling depression that S. felt had roots in his adolescence but increased in middle age to a totality that he knew could signal his own demise, by his own hand. He had responsibly explored every sanctioned option in an attempt to gain some relief, without success. He then decided to follow his friend's legally problematic advice to explore work with MDMA and this, as can be seen from the outcomes he achieved, came with success. For such an individual, and there are many, to be denied access to the healing potential of this medicine in the absence of any effective course of action is, in our view, the denial of a basic human right.

I had run out of options. After ten years of psychoanalysis, my depressions were getting worse. They had begun in my teens, a night here or there where my 'Black Dog,' as Winston Churchill called it, would come to visit. I would be up all night, numbing myself with the television set. The next day would be the hardest. I would be down the 'hole', unable to get out of bed. I would lie there, often with the room blacked out until the cloud lifted, and I could finally enter the world again. These depressive moments, I used to call them my 'de-compressions', would happen every few weeks or so, and for years they would only last maybe a day or two. But in my forties, they suddenly got worse. What had been a day here or there became days or even weeks. Now, the episodes turned into extended bouts which could last over a period of months.

What was this like? There would be days when I could not get out of bed. It's difficult to explain to someone who has not experienced it. This is not sadness or distress. It is an agonising despair without any release. It grips you in a vise and will not let you go. It is unrelenting, vicious, and without relief. It is this which drives you to suicide. Or did me. I never made an actual attempt to kill myself. But I knew with an absolute certainty that I would do so. To live in such anguish was not an option.

I eventually reached out to a friend in London, and he introduced me to the use of what I call the 'medicine'.

I remember the first session so very clearly. It was a home in an upscale neighbourhood. The man who would facilitate and attend to me during the treatment had a gentle and reassuring demeanour. He sat several feet from me. We spoke for a while. I told him I had been struggling with depression. I also said that I suspected that the depressions were borne of a childhood trauma that had happened when I was about eleven years old. It involved me being beaten by someone who was supposed to have been looking after me. I had been discussing the beating for months in therapy but without any relief from symptoms of the trauma. He advised that I just let the medicine do its work.

I took the first of two doses and lay back on the couch. At first, nothing happened. I just lay there and waited. And then waited. I kept thinking I felt different and wondered if the medicine's effect was subtle. I was starting to think this was yet another dead end. And then the medicine arrived. It washed over me, and I was dropped into a pool of pleasure. It was like a serotonin bath. The first words I spoke were, "Thank God, oh, thank you." It was the first relief I had felt from the vice grip of despair I had felt for years.

Then, the work began.

Almost unbidden, the trauma arrived. I was back in time, eleven years old, and I was reliving what I had gone through. I was being beaten. But this time, I could remember it properly, all the emotions, the thoughts that raced through my head, the fear, the thought that I was going to die, and that this was happening at the hands of someone who was supposed to love me. I had always remembered the event and had always known that it had affected me, and even cobbled me. But now, I was able to remember all of it, the entirety of the experience, in all its fullness. I writhed on the bed as my body remembered trying to ward off the blows. I grunted from the remembered pain. But throughout, I was still being bathed in the pleasure provided by the medicine. It made remembering the trauma possible. And then, suddenly, the trauma melted away. Like a tight Gordian knot unravelled, this event which had tattooed itself into my psychic skin, was dissolved.

I went back for a couple of more sessions, where I was able to explore what had happened to me a little more. I discovered a few other aspects of the experience but the most significant impact happened in that first session.

Since then, I have not had a day of depression. I have had sadness, challenges, and difficult times but none of the despair that I had lived with all those years. I have started a new career with the beginnings of real success. My marriage is so much better, and I am able to connect with people around me in new and substantial ways.

I am so grateful to have found this treatment. I don't know what would have been if I had not.

The poignancy of S.'s last sentence exists as an indictment of our present, and to our view, wholly inadequate system of relieving trauma. That our culture has deliberately failed to acknowledge the healing potential of MDMA is fundamentally inexcusable. To become the innocent victim of an act perpetrated upon us, and to have to carry that toxic event forward into our lives as trauma caught and held within us without real hope of release, is to cruelly compound the impact of the original traumatic event.

The prohibition of this medicine has inhibited research into its healing potential. This, once again, demonstrates the pernicious influence of fear-based decisions on our lives.

• • •

Snatch a pill. I was so guilty of that; I was so guilty of that.

Once Blind but Now Can See.

The following excerpts are from a discursive conversation following an MDMA session, and give some flavour of the eternal vigilance necessary for an individual in recovery to stay on the straight and narrow. From a life of mindlessness characterised by addiction to drugs and sex, here we see a man humbled by his past as he discusses aspects of the mindfulness he brings to his daily life following his medicine work. This is true for all of us; the work does not stop when the medicine stops affecting us. The medicine work is a gift, and then the real work starts.

Feelings? I don't think I had ever felt them. Usually, I would turn and run. When I was allowed to embrace it through the medicine, just allow them, OK, I just walked through it. That's extraordinary. It shows me what I need to do when I leave and just walk through it or let it go or at least to be aware of it; ideally just let it go.

It's authentic, MDMA. I think that's the word I'm looking for. There's nothing distorted. If anything, it's clarified. It's a very interesting, interesting process. I have no desire to ever use it recreationally, zero.

Yeah, it's interesting. I know it's helped a lot of people. That's what's crazy too. Think about it; we're kind of wired these days to be desensitised to everything, particularly our own pain, and it's just a search for instant gratification we're all in. And it's hard to get in touch with any real underlying emotions. It's fucking crazy out there. When you've got some crazy in there, and you're trying to get crazy fixed out there, it ain't gonna work.

Snatch a pill. I was so guilty of that; I was so guilty of that. That's the way I ran my life with narcotics, and it was crazy. I almost killed myself. Now, I don't take any of that shit. I take Ashwagandha every day for mood. It's great. It's one of the oldest Indian herbs ever used medicinally, and it's for our mood. It's a natural antidepressant medication. Ashwagandha is wonderful. I take a GABA every day, high quality fish oils, good buffered Vitamin C to detoxify my body, and a few other things for my heart; we have got to take care of ourselves, eat smart. If I can avoid a pharmaceutical solution I will avoid it at all costs. It's fucking chemicals and crap. You take one, and you get a side effect, and you have to take something else to offset that. It's such a circus, it's not even funny.

When I was coming off narcotics…I was on Oxycontin for years, I fucked up my bowels so bad, because it is a very constipating drug. They constipate you, so after being on it for years, my digestive system was so screwed up. Then, when you come off, you get the runs something fierce. It seemed like years for me. I had just horrible screwed up bowels. It was horrible, horrible.

You know what? There's so much crazy dysfunction in our world today. You just look at the television. The shit they have on TV today; it's so fucking crazy.

One day in my house, there were nine females, my three daughters and their friends. I had to leave my own house; I couldn't stand it anymore! They're beautiful kids and wonderful children, but the oestrogen was just out of control. Even the flippin' cat is female.

If there is one good thing I've done right in my life, it is that once I fucked up, and I fucked up pretty good, I turned it around and realised what an awesome responsibility I have to those girls. Awesome opportunity to blow it. It doesn't take much to go either way. It's a trip every day. I will tell you that there are days when I just feel so inept as a father, it's not even funny. It's a lifelong journey; my daughters keep my feet pointed in the right direction.

You know, this shit running around in our heads? Being controlled by our fears. If I'm a present, stable father, there's a better chance that they'll learn by my example. Especially with girls, if you want them to have some decent self-esteem and make smart choices in life. My middle one is so smart; it's ridiculous. But she's not just brains, she's got a huge soul. Love emanates from that child. She's got some quirks and insecurities like we all do, but a good kid.

If I would have stayed on that path with narcotics and all of that shit, there is no way my kids would have been OK. I was on drugs from when they were born until my oldest was six; then, we separated. As far as divorces go, I could have had it a lot, lot worse. I was kicked out of the house multiple times for cheating in my marriage. I was terrified. I was not a good husband. I was terrified. I was just terrified of intimacy, still am terrified of intimacy.

My kids saw some of it. My oldest was probably affected the most. She's going to find her way out. The little one, it's too early to tell. She's going to be fine. She's flighty. She's very much like her mother, which is probably a good thing.

You know, I call them the tapes that we have running in our heads. It's the messaging we were given as very young people. We were given this message, whatever it is, that the world is fearful or the world is angry. We don't know what to do as children with that. We're sponges, so we suck this shit up and we suck this chaos into our psyches. What I've come to realise is that this is the human condition. Everybody's got something, I don't care who you are, you've got something.

There's pain, there's grief, there's joy, and disappointment. If you're human, you're going to experience those emotions. Most people don't know how to process through those feelings. I didn't. I didn't. Why do you think I was acting out in my marriage all the time? I shouldn't say I behaved in a predatory way. There are plenty of willing, broken 'other women' participants out there that were just as broken as I was, and we found each other. You're seeking a solution in sex, and it's fucking crazy.

Well, I know what it is now, I mean just complete fear of intimacy with women centred on a huge lack of self-esteem in myself.

From an unconscious life predicated by a personality formed on his behalf by others, this individual can now see his past behaviour for what it was. The first step was to bring the behaviour into consciousness, take responsibility for it, experience and examine it and, with resolve, to take steps every day to ameliorate the damage he had wrought. From many years of being addicted to drugs that are potentially more powerful than heroin, drugs manufactured and freely sold by the medical-industrial complex, his body has paid a terrible price. Understanding this, he has investigated the healing potential of centuries-old natural remedies, using herbs, oils, and vitamins to bring his body into alignment with the capacity for love he can now feel for his daughters. This is a true expression of 'duty of care'.

• • •

One is invited to engage with a deep internal energetic force.

M. B.

If one harboured any lingering doubts about the true nature of the action of this medicine vis a vis its public identity as a 'party drug', observing the progression of this individual's many medicine sessions would put them all to rest. When M. came for his consultation, it was clear from his frantic presentation of the byzantine details of his life that this man was in deep, deep trouble. Customarily, the medicine will unfold traumas in reverse chronological order, the most recent first, and there was so much traumatic material in his biography that it was not possible to even venture a guess as to what might emerge. He took the first dose of MDMA and within twenty minutes lay on his side facing me with a look of absolute horror on his face; he had leapfrogged every terrible thing that had happened over fifty years and encountered his mother on the first day of his life.

I first came to this work in 2012, through exhaustive searching and the help of a few generous people. I had known that I had PTSD for several decades, but had no clear perspective of any conceivable cure. Let me be the first to say that working with MDMA can be difficult, requiring some perseverance to overcome, but then quickly transforms into an extraordinary sense of awe and optimism. I had done countless years of therapy in multiple directions and, in time, sadly had submitted to a life of surreal resignation. At my lowest point, I had purchased a handgun and was trying to write the script for my own demise. Alternately, I considered hospitalisation and had gone through many frustrated therapists and useless medications.

I arrived at a first with an MDMA attendant telling stories of ten years of cult life in my twenties, abruptly cut short by a kidnapping and illegal intervention that had not resulted in any renouncement of personal convictions, but rather that drove a permanent wedge between my family and myself and hardened my will. I also had earlier history as a runaway from home in my teens, and the course of my life was shaped much earlier by a very abusive home life. The systemic nature of PTSD builds upon previous traumas until, like rising waters in a dam, it spills over into one's everyday awareness as a replay of unresolved painful memories and a dissociative numbing effect. Disorganisation, depression, disbelief, and desperation are common hallmarks. There is, literally, no way out, and maybe just as bad, no one seems to know the answers.

And then, one arrives at the point of contact with MDMA in a therapeutic setting. This is very important to understand: There is nothing recreational about this encounter. The setting is quiet and internally focused. One is guided to engage with a deep internal energetic force. If possible, one finds the means to let go. Only metaphors can describe the grace and empathic qualities that open before you as you experience vistas of promise. The obvious goal being release and relief from a world of hurt going back, in my case, an entire lifetime.

I am very much in agreement with the thesis of the "unexperienced experience." I had spent, literally, decades trying to uncover the sources of my anxiety and dissociation through various therapies. My subconscious explored endlessly in nightmarish dreams. I always came close but had no actual resolutions. The problem, I believe, was that the original traumatic film had jammed, cut, and spliced, and I had NO recollection of actual events in real time. I could never summon the dark memories deeply enough, nor could I locate the undamaged self from my beginnings. This is where MDMA retrieves the lost footage from a long-lost archive and allows the viewer to ease into full experience for the very first time.

I had been a typical teenager—pursuing cars, guitars, and girls—and, I felt, was a part of a wonderful generation of seekers. I became interested in spirituality, leading to my quasi-cult years. In this spiritual community, I felt gifted, and through extensive meditation could achieve and maintain a state of deep peace and absorption. I spoke at public events about these experiences and associated with many young people deeply committed to a disciplined spiritual lifestyle. It was a time of deep peace and inner wonder.

Somewhere into those years, my life was violently interrupted by an attack by anti-cult zealots and mercenaries. This was the 1970s, right after Jim Jones and Charles Manson, and the public was very frightened by charismatic movements. I endured the deprogramming ordeal of six weeks as a prisoner in locked and guarded confines. I grew withdrawn, mistrusting, and angry until after about a year and half, I imploded. In one single moment, I collapsed into an anxiety ridden, socially inhibited, basket case. It was so abrupt and complete that I never recovered. My body was constantly re-experiencing an assault from within. I became riddled with uncontrollable nerves; my senses retreated into a world of bizarre dissociation in which nothing looked or felt real anymore. The loss was staggering. I couldn't look another human being in the eye without spiralling into paranoia. It was a complete and total loss of equanimity and stopped all ambition in its tracks. I felt under siege from every angle; the world went dark. What had seemed like a marvellous world had turned inside out for me, and, suddenly, I was living in the realm of damaged souls. This went on for, literally, thirty years.

During this time, I met my wife and we started and raised a family. I survived as a self-employed carpenter-contractor with complete lack of psychological and physical self-regulation and became a workaholic and eventually an alcoholic. As the years progressed, I would face numerous defeats and obstacles that only served to deepen my sense of despair. Desperately seeking relief in 2010, I contracted with a high-tech neuro-feedback outfit claiming to cure anxiety syndromes and similar nervous system disorders. This intensive pseudo-scientific experience completely backfired and plunged me into an even deeper state of disorientation. I lost 15 percent of my body weight, and my sleep was reduced to one or two hours per night with rampant nightmares. After that, I went on a determined mission to find help and tried every new conceivable mental health avenue at great expense. This led to my last gasp of searching, until I came in contact with MDMA in 2012.

My progress has been hard to measure in this work, I will freely admit. I have continued with determination and reverence, because nothing has ever come close to accomplishing what MDMA therapy has offered. I have been regularly involved for over three years.

I am certain, through the illumination of this work, that the origins of my problems were simple but devastating childhood developmental trauma. A child abandoned and neglected absorbs so much negativity that the effect is one of passive abuse. I have experienced specific deliverance from these complex symptoms through direct experience under the benevolent influence of this medicine. By re-encountering very early memories in the MDMA state, I have seen my identity crises unfold, and I've been released from their dark and destructive effects.

In describing this work, there is sometimes a tendency to proselytise. I wish the reader to grasp the sheer miraculous benefits that are possible by engaging with this powerful ally, MDMA, and at the same time, shed any notion of a fashionable trend. Despite abstract battles and dark passages, MDMA becomes one's best friend internally and restores the lost sensibilities of trust, wonder, and appreciation. This becomes an accomplishment of monumental proportions for sufferers of PTSD. In the end, one's internal prison is slowly dissolved, and the return to simplicity is overwhelming. After one session, I came home and woke the next morning happily daydreaming away like a carefree child. I had not been able to relax to this degree for over fifty years. It was astonishing and brought me to tears.

I try with some difficulty to explain the workings of MDMA to a rational mind. It has an ability to restructure our emotional perspective to such a degree that we are won over to a completely new reality. This state creates a deep realignment, allowing us to receive gifts from a seemingly magical world. Afterward, the effects of these gifts can remain intact permanently. In its ability to return us to a pure state of being, healing simply happens. In my opinion, I can say that MDMA is quite possibly the most benign substance on earth.

I hope to continue with this work, until I can function fully again as a conscious, creative, and caring human being with all emotional and perceptional functions restored. As the future unfolds, I can think of nothing more rewarding than to help others cross these same bridges themselves. I am extremely grateful to the attendants for providing a safe and secure environment for many like myself to find lasting relief from a previously intractable disorder.

Early on in this work, I was repeatedly brought to deep concern for my immediate family members and my son; he had been a serious drug addict for over ten years. My wife and I had spent tens of thousands of dollars on rehabs, halfway houses, lawyers, clinics, and the like. He had lost countless friends to overdose, car crashes, and suicide. He was, for all intents, a lost cause, ending up frequently in jail or ERs. At one point, my wife asked, "Do you think MDMA could help him?" I said it could not hurt and arranged for him to conduct three MDMA sessions in the same manner I had undergone.

The result was nothing short of miraculous. My son became a transformed individual. In one session, he called me to say, "I had never known there was another train of thought available (other than drug addiction)." Somehow, in a deep MDMA state, he could see the path out of his own personal hell. The other two sessions allowed further opening to major changes in his life. He went on to work with iboga (once only) and kicked his habit completely. Not only is he still clean to this day, he now has a career, is buying a house, and is involved in a committed relationship. There could not be a more bright and inspired outcome to his once tragic story. I owe a debt of gratitude to the attendants and MDMA for saving his life.

M.'s slow progress in this work is not atypical of someone who experienced developmental trauma at the hands of their parents every day of their lives. One time, he was with his mother in the woods, when they saw and heard a pack of wolves on a ridge; "Perhaps, I will leave you here for the wolves," she said. This was not humour; this was mother. His lack of speed in the work has been matched by his steadiness and his unrelenting resolve, wherein every setback has been met with courage and continuance. He constantly observed the workings of his mind during the session and would often describe the action of his huge resistance in real time as it was occurring. An example from his first session: He said that, at one point, "The sirens were beckoning," wanting him to enjoy the medicine more fully but immediately his fine, rational mind stepped in to say, "Don't be a bloody fool, this is not happening," whereupon the sirens retreated. He clearly saw from experience and understanding that resistance is always the mind's doing.

On various occasions over numerous sessions, he has said such bon mots as, "I see vistas of promise." "Pain is resistance," and "I can feel the medicine wants to heal me." These spontaneous expressions of his internal process result from a keen spiritual interest in figuring out the mechanism-of-action that enables such true understanding of ourselves, and they have kept his nose to the golden grindstone of his psyche's machinations. The medicine always has our best interests at heart and is congenitally incapable of deceiving us or taking us in the wrong direction. It's enormous but its only role is to move us toward wholeness and coherence, and as his work progressed, M, could not but share the benefits he had experienced with his beloved son, who had been MIA for many years because of his heroin addiction. His testimony follows.

• • •

I was out of all resources and ideas.

B. B.

I knew a lot about B. from working with his father, who had always expressed great love for his son, with recollections of adventures they had enjoyed with fun and laughter while he was growing up. As the father was changed from his own medicine work, he listened to his wife and became able to consider the possibility of including B., leading to a consultation and then three sessions. During the first of these, the street-talk had me feeling as if I were with B. among a group of addicts, with profanities and drug-world slang. During the second, we sat by the window smoking cigarettes. I told him I had never taken heroin and asked if there were any similarities between it and the MDMA he was now experiencing. He thought about it a few moments and said, yes, they were similar in their ability to enable us to feel relaxed and without fear. I remarked that, unlike the addictive drug heroin, this medicine would not come back tomorrow and make any demands at all of him, and this enabled him to relax.

I would like to introduce myself as a grateful, blessed, and honoured man, willing to share my experience, strength, and hope. I was, once, someone you might call an addict; I have what they call a disease. My mission in life, however, was to stop using drugs. I am not huge on AA or NA (as they are the only accepted kinds of treatment in the eyes of many). I believe everyone has at least one addiction (of course, coffee and heroin are completely different), but there is a chemical dependence that most people have. I am a recovering heroin addict. I hope this testimony may serve as an example of how MDMA treatment can accomplish what the typical counselling could not (at least, for me).

Being labelled an addict is a tough pill to swallow, no pun intended. I had been through every kind of facility. Roughly eight to ten years (off and on) of programmes, counselling, and psychiatry. Thirty, sixty, or even ninety days didn't work. Toward the end, I went to a one-year programme and was even a house manager at one point!

Looking back, that place had all the elements and just the right amount of freedom one could ask for in a structured programme. I managed for a while, but like many other programmes, there were always a few bad apples that were still using or drinking on weekends. For example, my roommate (and best friend at this place) was doing dope, but I could not rat someone else out. After he got kicked out, a month later, I decided to up and walk away.

Now, this was from a place where some real healing and sobriety could've been reachable, but basically, I was not ready to face life, the mistakes, and problems of my past. I came to a point where I really realised I had to fix my life, sad that it took so long. Every day was a constant battle to find the money and the dope. I walked through the ghettos of major cities; many, I was lucky to walk out of. I have made multiple trips to jail, five different facilities to be exact, and stayed six months the last time.

I still wanted to STOP using. I had wanted to stop, or to find the next course of action. Addicts are relentless and crafty chameleons as they try and blend in with society, and certain people (me) who are given the title of an addict or dope-fiend develop lies to cover tracks. When in full addiction, you are in constant NEED of something that is gone so fast. I knew better, but nothing ever worked, because I was not able to FEEL certain emotions anymore.

In my opinion, even the state facilities have the same lectures, ideas, books, and tools for being successful. I learned a whole lot at each place and most helped me to better understand addiction. However, I was still stuck in a revolving door, having been in and out of jail, programmes, sober livings, you name it. If it was a drug course, methadone programme, or twelve-step, I'd done it. I'm sorry to say it did not matter where in the country I was or how severe my charges were, I just didn't commit until I was ready. I was in what I called the Dark Side, which is a mindset I adopted when using.

I strongly feel my story could help someone who has any addiction that they want to be rid of. My past has been rough, and I've been so hard-headed. Ultimately, I am a good example of someone who has not only been to hell and back but almost gave up on fighting all together. I'm glad to say that this method became available to me. I had been told by a good friend who had been searching, that this treatment had helped them greatly. My father introduced me to someone who offered it.

I must stay anonymous, but my story doesn't need a name to

understand the importance or impact. This would be regarding the experience of MDMA, which I call the root, the ONE, or the source. This was done in the company of one who was happy to listen to my most inner problems, doubts, and past stuff that I just couldn't let go of.

When I found out about this treatment using MDMA, my initial thought was how are you supposed to treat an addict with more drugs? I had tried this same substance before but in a party setting. This time it was different. It opened a gate to experience a feeling that I did not know I could feel anymore. It took me several sessions with good intentions and the best company one could ask for.

Lying by myself and in the hands of a seasoned, educated, and just all-around noble person, with safe surroundings, I found the answers I was seeking. My mind was clear and the comforting light inside of me was warm and forgiving of my wrongs. It was like one part of me could not get over the guilt and suffering that I had caused. I wanted to get in touch with me, the person I knew before the dope.

I'm a sincere, loyal, and trusting person. I'm happy to say this part of me is alive and well again. I needed to get in touch with the real me that loves to have fun and to laugh, that has good intentions and cares about the people closest to me. I found my experience with MDMA to be priceless. It was completely different with my eyes closed and peeling back internal layers that I could not channel before. In the third session, I had an experience where I finally felt happy (which was nice for a change) and confident that I could follow through on a promise to myself and to THE ONE, THE SOURCE, MY HIGHER POWER, whatever you may call it.

That started a chain of events that landed me on the path to what I would have never thought possible. Now, it has been four or more years since my last trip. I finally have my family back in my life; my girlfriend and I just had our one-year anniversary. I have a career that I am good at, and I have kept for three years and still going strong. But can you guess what I don't have the desire or need for? Dope!

I am not saying this is a cure for addiction, but for me it was, in a sense, because it allowed me to believe again. I felt the feeling of love and hope. I felt ways that I had not been able to for years, and had the drive to follow through with my decision to defeat my addiction.

Sitting with B. over three sessions, one could sense the knife-edge he was on, and for all the progress he was making in the work, he still had the monkey on his back. His parents had already looked into the possibility of ibogaine, an African root-bark that has a robust reputation as a medicine that can interrupt addiction to give the addict time to get themselves together. One advocate has called it, "Chapter 11 for addicts." This seemed to be exactly what B. needed, and after his third session with MDMA, he submitted himself to a week in an ibogaine clinic. This intervention successfully completed his recovery from a decade-long career as an addict and the return to the normal function he describes as 'blessed' in his testimony.

◦ ◦ ◦

It's a gift that keeps unpacking itself.

Jack L.

Jack is a forthright, competent, and successful individual who might appear to have the world at his command. Yet, he had been struck by how much shame he carried, and a spontaneous incident of feeling this intensely led to a palpable release. Following the realisation of the power and depth of his shame, he felt that something had lifted and this unsolicited, spontaneous, and organic event demonstrates the potential of the psyche to release even without the influence of MDMA. In this instance, the spontaneous release was unmediated by medicine, an unsolicited but nevertheless welcome event. We are at pains to be forthright about any demonstration of this extraordinary, in-built ability of the body to heal itself.

A couple of years ago, my life seemed to be getting more and more constricted. I found that I was getting in my own way more and more, and I couldn't figure out why. I had this sense that I always got in my own way a little bit, but I was getting in my own way more than I ever had. I don't really remember how this came up, but it became clear that there was something that had happened to me when I was very young that I wanted to avoid, and the way I avoided it was I wouldn't admit that it had happened.

It was essentially an abusive mother who was emotionally unstable. I think now she had what they call...something about dysphoric syndrome. It's PMS that is so hellacious that the woman becomes a completely different person, almost a split personality. My mother had it. Some mornings, I would wake up to kisses and hugs, and some mornings, I'd wake up to screaming and slapping. I never knew which it was going to be.

From that, I guess I learned that there was something wrong with me, and that I brought this on myself somehow. I carried this deep, deep sense of shame, and I didn't even really know what it was. I couldn't name it. When it became clear that it was shame and that I really did have to finally acknowledge the consequences this had in my life, I was just overwhelmed, and I didn't know what to do.

My dear old friend, Carl, with whom I have just reconnected with after a long time, started telling me about this work that he had done, and it was something that he had to tell me, because we had been out of touch for twenty years. He and his boyfriend, now husband, came to my wedding twenty-one years ago, and then he dropped from sight shortly after that, because he was traumatised and just couldn't function. He was telling me about how he'd got through that and really come to a completely different place that he didn't think he was going to get to again. I said, "That sounds like it's for me." He told me all about it, and I thought, "How soon can I meet this chap? How soon can I do it?" It wasn't very long; it was only a couple of weeks.

I think I was so primed to let that out of my life and let the consequences of it out of my life. Late that summer, I was out for a walk near my house, and because it's in the country, I was by myself. I remember feeling this flattening, overwhelming sense of shame. I had some realisation, finally, that it hadn't been my fault, and it was a revelation. It was like a printing press had been lifted from my chest. There was a completely different physical sensation that I was aware of. That primed me for this. It primed me for being able to really unlock what this was about and release it.

When I came to see the attendant, I felt instantly reassured. Everything that my friend had told me was true. I met a nice, kind man who I could obviously trust with my life, essentially. I felt completely comfortable doing that, and he explained to me in wonderful detail what the medicine was going to do, how long it would take to have an effect, how long the effect would last, and what it might be like. He reassured me that no matter what happened, he would stay with me and attend to me. I remember that was the word he used, "attend." I felt completely safe, and I laid down on the couch, and he was in the chair. I took this stuff, and I was relaxed, and everything felt fine. I remember we were talking a little bit and having a conversation, and it began to come on very quickly. I was aware of it; it was quite dramatic, and I could just sort of felt the vortex opening up. It felt very welcoming; I didn't have any hesitation of any kind. I knew that it would take me in.

It started to come on, and I was completely comfortable with it. I knew that it was just going to completely take me away. It did. I lost all sense of myself as a separate being, which is something I'm pretty comfortable with from a lot of meditation for many years. I just went with it, and it was so comfortable. I remember hearing, it was a warm day; it was a sunny, lovely beautiful day; there was a breeze. I remember hearing the windows were open. I remember hearing the breeze and the leaves rustling. I remember hearing the children in the schoolyard playing, and none of it was separate from me. I was all those things. I was still me, but I was all of those things as well. There was no other; I was everything. I was everything, and everything was me.

It lasted five hours. I felt like I'd had the most wonderful sleep of my life. I felt like I'd just been born again, but born the right way! It wasn't as dramatic when I came back, of course, though I felt like some more of that load had been lifted. It's a gift that keeps unpacking itself. For months and months afterward, I felt this ease of being that I had never known in my whole life.

People have always told me that I was comfortable in my own skin, and I guess, based on what people see, to some degree I was. I probably gave the impression of being comfortable to a greater degree than I was, because I had learned how to hide that shame pretty well. All of a sudden, I was living the image that I think I was projecting. I was authentically connected to that sense of kind of a commander who could take charge of things and not in a way that felt overpowering. It was just that I fully inhabited myself.

I thought of a phrase that Timothy Leary said, which was, "The archives of the unconscious are inexhaustible." And that's really what it seemed like. There's a certain detachment to it. There's a connection, but there's an emotional detachment. It doesn't feel threatening, but you can fully experience it. So, when I say, "fully inhabited," it had always felt like something was missing before that. I was missing something.

That's what shame does, of course. It makes you feel like, "I'm broken. There's something wrong with me. I can't function like a normal human being, and that is an option that will never be open to me," and that just went away. There was a great relief at first, but over time, as I stopped living and feeling that way, the memory of it faded too. It all seemed to fade into the background. I can remember being that way. I can remember feeling that way, but it's only a memory now. It has nothing to do with who I am.

I finally fully inhabited myself. I am so grateful to the attendant and to that substance and to whoever invented that substance, or synthesised it. I think it's a therapeutic tool that is invaluable, and I look forward to a time when the hysteria and paranoia about the abuse potential can be put in perspective to the unbelievably therapeutic potential that that substance contains. Because it would be a crime for what's happened over the last thirty years since MDMA was criminalised because people were just using it for fun. It would be horrible if that continued much longer, because there's too much need for this. There's so much trauma in this country, not to mention all the thousands and thousands of returning veterans who are suffering from PTSD.

This is a way out; I mean this is a way past that, rather than just giving them a Band-Aid and a pair of crutches. I mean, that's the therapeutic approach now pretty much; it's very stop-gap. This is something that can just release it, take it away.

Until we have experienced the action of MDMA and its ability to sweetly bring us to a deeper understanding of our psyches and by extension of ourselves, we cannot know this medicine's potential to benefit us. For too many years my own understanding of the action of MDMA was that it made you feel good. But therapeutic? Yet, we can see from Jack's testimony, where he recounts the 'flattening, overwhelming' sense of shame that he became aware of during a walk in the country, that the body's ability to allow release from trauma is entirely natural. The spontaneous eruption of symptoms in the form of flashbacks or insights that may be troubling in ordinary life, is, in fact, the ongoing project of the body to release itself from the burden it carries, with or without our active involvement. This focused work with MDMA, however, gives us the finest opportunity to reliably create and maintain the optimal condition for such releases to occur at a time and place of our choosing.

* * *

I am so thankful for having been a part of it.

Harish.

Reflecting his nervousness about the legal implications, Harish requested we first meet in a public park like Cold War spooks, and we subsequently went on to have a number of preparatory meetings to explain the work with MDMA. It seemed mysterious to him, impossible even, but it eventually became comprehensible enough for him to commit to work with the medicine. As we were finalising this testimony, he wrote, "I feel I was on the same page as you when we first met. I was so eager for you to get back in touch with me in the first place. I remember being 100 percent in-line with your point of view. I remember you mentioning to me the people you worked with and studied with. I shared how I had encountered the works of some of the same people, and how I had read a lot more than I had experienced. I felt like I got what was behind the work, at least intellectually. I was all in. I was just scared. Hence, needing to meet with you multiple times. It was mostly to get comfortable. That's all. There was no doubt or trouble understanding for me. Only fear. That little thing."

Even as he took full advantage in-session of the MDMA condition to dwell fruitfully on troubling aspects of his childhood, and referencing his robust meditation practice, the sense of mystery remained. He writes, "The feelings of mysteriousness and impossibility sure did crop up after doing the work however, but in the best possible way." It was as if he was saying, "Really?" to what the medicine brought forth, not in doubt of the facts but in awe and wonder as to how this could have been accomplished so handily.

We feel the same way.

The work is always mysterious. I am never quite sure what is going to come out of it. Before doing it the first time, I was just ending a stressful teaching job and transitioning into taking physics courses at a local university. I remember the great feelings of fear and uncertainty I had making this transition. I was also at this time desperate to have a relationship with a woman.

The MDMA experience, itself, was very gentle. I felt very safe in the space. I felt very comfortable lying on the couch with the blindfold on, ready to receive the experience. It comes on so gently. It is just a feeling of feeling good all around. With all the good feelings, before I had a chance to realise it, I was in another state of consciousness. I can't really describe how exactly it is different, but it is different. The most important moment I can remember during that experience was when suddenly, in an instant, my father came into my mind, and my heart opened up completely. It was profound. I knew what I had learned right then and there. That my father feels the same way that I feel. He is a being capable of emotions like me. He feels sadness, anger, and fear just like me. I am like him, and he is like me.

The other important thing to note about the experience was the importance of having someone present. It was so comforting and safe to know that there was someone else there. This was most important when coming down from the most intense peaks of the experience. It can feel quite sudden coming down to more of a baseline from these peaks. It is in these moments where I needed to hold a hand. It was so helpful through those moments. It often only lasted a second or two and then I was fine again. Having someone there, when the whole experience had run its course, was so important too. Being able to talk and sit with someone at such a special time.

The situation with my father is forever different. There is something deep down. My love for him that got reawakened. I speak to him differently now. I speak to him like a person. I used to speak to him the way my mother spoke to him, treating him as unintelligent and not capable. But I can tell the difference now. I can tell when my heart closes to him and I go back to this old way of being with him. I can tell when my mom yells at him. I can feel what it does to my heart. I feel like some deep connection to my father and my own manhood has been restored.

The work has given me many other insights and realisations. Such as to what it feels like to really enjoy life and be happy. What it feels like to shamelessly take off my shirt. How to be more kind and gentle with myself. How to show my genuine anger to someone. How to love myself. How to value my voice and opinions. I credit it for opening me up to swimming, running, and martial arts. I credit it for healing some sort of rift between me and my sister. I credit it for opening me up to a woman who has shown me so much love and kindness.

The work has been such a gift. I am so thankful for having been a part of it.

The most important factor in approaching the medicine work is our decision to show up for ourselves; it is absolutely key. This medicine work is interactive, requiring our focus and attention, whereas our relationship to most medicines is entirely passive, following the "Take two of these and call me in the morning" model. There is nothing for us to do but take the medicine and wait for it to take effect. Not so with MDMA; the medicine opens us to the contents of our psyche, and it is then our job to seize upon these revelations and engage with them. Essentially, we are interacting with ourselves, and by so doing, we can engage with many aspects of our personality that may be obscure to us. In Harish's case, this engagement included an intense recalibration of his relationship with his father.

Harish writes, "The lessons from the work are still present with me today. After a lifetime of self-judgement and trying to correct things about myself, the work gave me a chance to really experience feeling OK. Feeling good. That there is nothing wrong with me. There is nothing to correct. That it is OK to love myself and accept myself how I am right now. I don't have to work more at something else before I get to do that." His sense of gratitude is echoed by many of the individuals undertaking this work.

● ● ●

I could not imagine this happening before I started the work.

Frank I.

Frank's enduring struggle with resistance is wholly characteristic of working with the developmental trauma from which he suffers. In-session, his agitation is expressed by frequent bouts of sitting up with his face in a contorted, vivid expression of the 'ache' that is the major part of his psychic life. Rilke asks that we "go toward the difficult," and after sitting up, as he lay down again to face this personal hell, he would say things that I took note of: "Shaming was the go-to tactic of my family;" "I would've gladly given up all the accolades I got for my school work for a single hug;" and, "I think I was resented as a foetus." This mulling of experiences as they emerged would continue, until it became unbearable, and he simply could not do it any longer. Then, he would sit up again, eyes open, his face the mask of tragedy. This is work.

In the mid-1980s, I had a couple of experiences with MDMA,

before it was made illegal. I felt a sense of calmness and bliss that I've tried to recapture ever since. Years later, when I started reading about MDMA and PTSD, I just identified with the PTSD symptoms even though I haven't been to war, I haven't been raped, and I haven't had that kind of abuse or incident in my past. I just identified with the symptoms, and I believed that working with MDMA in a controlled, therapeutic setting would help. Although I've gained a lot from traditional therapy, I felt like I could just talk to my regular therapist for decades and not get as deep as I needed to go.

I had no idea what I was getting into, but I kinda liked that. My attendant had prepared a couch to lie on and had set out water and juice. I quickly felt at home in the room and with him. I took 125 mg of MDMA, put on my eyeshade, and lay back.

We began shortly before noon, and the session (with a 75 mg boost about ninety minutes after we started) lasted over five hours. The transitions into and out of my heightened state were extraordinarily subtle. There was never a "boing!" moment when I felt it kick in; there was only a simple "aha" moment when I realised the journey had already begun.

Soft chamber music played. For the duration, my attendant never left me alone, except for his own bathroom breaks or to get me juice or food. I felt safe, and he seemed comfortable and committed to his role.

Although I had brought a notebook in which to write, my attendant encouraged me to keep my eyes closed and just allow the journey. He volunteered to write down anything I dictated to him. Over the next five hours, there were stretches of silence, but also *a lot* of thoughts I wanted to remember. He ended up filling nineteen pages.

It was great to be able to lie down and see where my thoughts went, but it was much deeper than that. I'm very grateful the attendant took notes, because when I read what I said during that session, I was struck by how wise some of the things were and how aware I was of who I was, what had happened to me, and the path to freedom. It was as if the medicine had facilitated a deep and revealing conversation with myself. Especially about the role that shame has played in my life, and the myriad ways I was mistreated and neglected by my family growing up, both by my parents and by my older siblings.

I felt completely safe during the session, and for two weeks afterwards, I felt a sort of natural high. Then, I went for a walk one night, and I just crashed. I suddenly realised some very dark stuff about my mom, and that, if I had followed the path and rules she had wanted me to follow, I'd be dead now. I knew I needed to do a lot more work, and I committed to doing so. I've had twelve sessions so far over two years.

As I continued the work, I got very much in touch with my resistance, the part of me that didn't want to go to the dark place and that blocked it with relentless vigour. I found that combining a little psilocybin with the MDMA has helped me go deeper.

For me, MDMA has often had this wonderful maternal feeling. There's a nice sort of hug to it. The first time I added a little psilocybin, I suddenly heard this very male voice inside of me say in a powerful, but not critical way, "Man up!" I just looked at that and said, "Whoa! Where did this come from?" I realised the psilocybin talks to me in a different way. I think it has helped strengthen my ego, and it has also taken me to much darker places. It's like they're this male/female team. There's a kind of rigour I feel under the psilocybin that the MDMA doesn't have. There's a comforting feeling I get from the MDMA that the psilocybin doesn't have. Together, it's been a kind of miraculous work.

After a while, I started wanting to come in to sessions with a specific intention. Sometimes, the intentions surprised me, but I've learned to listen to myself more and more. Once, although I had come up with some "uplifting" intentions, I realised the one I *really* wanted to explore was, "I want to tell my oldest brother to 'Fuck off!'" (In reality, my oldest brother had been dead for over a decade, but I still heard his critical and demeaning voice in my head, especially whenever I began feeling good about myself.) I was thinking, "Well, that's not a very warm touchy-feely intention," but I decided to trust it was the intention I needed to go with.

There was a strength I had in that session that I'd never experienced before. I got in touch with a beautiful anger, a delicious, "Fuck you!" It was also the only time in the sessions I've had so far where I got to a place of deep bliss. I repeatedly let go of my resistance, this ache I carry around in me, which is both a psychological but also physical ache; a kind of tension I carry that I have extreme trouble letting go of. In this session, I just kept letting go over and over. Effortlessly. It was wonderful.

I was in that blissful place for a few weeks. Then, I developed some medical problems (an appendectomy and complications), and the hospital treated me with such coldness and even a dangerous neglect that my PTSD came back hard. By the time the problems ended, I had lost touch with the blissful feelings I had. But I had the memory, which is wonderful to have. In the four sessions I've had since then, I came in with the hope I would recapture that bliss, knowing, of course, that you can't chase after it. I hope I will end up there again someday. I'm also aware that there's a level of magic to what happened that time. You can make room for magic, but you can never force it to happen.

My work "under the influence" has shown me that it's resistance, not wounds, that prevents the deepest healing. In my most recent session, my intention was "to see what was on the other side," to stop hiding parts of myself from myself. The result was my most intense session so far. I went to a place of primal horror and fear, an almost-consuming terror, an infantile place where I felt all alone in an unsafe world. I've seen these places from a distance in the past, but this was the first time I fully allowed myself to go there. I knew I could open my eyes and escape these feelings, but I chose to stay with them. It was challenging but very empowering. It speaks well of the work that I finally could surrender the way I could. I was ready to face this part of myself.

After sessions, I go home, rest, and type out the handwritten notes the attendant takes. It's been important to me to always leave a couple of days to rest after the session. There's all sorts of realisations and integration that bubble up for days and even weeks. The work also takes such a toll on me physically and emotionally that it's important to set aside two days after to just relax, go for a swim, and to share my journey with trusted friends.

I've compiled my notes into a notebook, which I look at regularly. I took it with me on the plane a couple of months ago. I started reading it, and at one point, I just put down the notebook, went to the bathroom, and started yelling into the mirror. I'm not sure where this rage came from, but it was so great that it came up. It was in me and needed to come out. I didn't feel overwhelmed by it, I knew I could stop, and it just felt great to be in connection with it. I could not imagine this happening before I started the work.

I've told some people about the work I'm doing, and often they've asked, "Oh, does it work?" If I look at it as a yes/no question, I can't say fully yes. I still have a lot of resistance. I still have a lot of ache. I certainly have all sorts of emotional issues to work on. However, the more I do the work, the more I see this is about healing and reconnection with the soul. I know myself better. I have more access to myself. I think I'm more open to people about who I am. I used to feel like a victim of my "ache." Now, on the best days, I see my relationship to my ache like I'm a kind and patient parent with a difficult child. I look forward to continuing the journey.

More from notes made during Frank's sessions: "I have to walk carefully to avoid landmines and barbed wire, the legacy of how it felt being a child." "I have spent my entire life trying to guess what crime I was convicted of." "I needed validation in such a brutal family," and, "My life has been a quest for validation in lieu of love." When such statements emerge unbidden from within the client under the benevolent influence of MDMA, we can only receive them as authentic expressions of the ongoing reality of their life experience. In a home environment like this, the child has no chance to see himself in any other way than that which is presented to him by the persons upon whom he is totally dependent, his mother and father. In Frank's case, this was exacerbated as he sees his trauma as the result of his terrified response not only to his parents but also to the larger environment that included three older siblings, especially two brothers.

The negative energy he internalised wholesale, believing himself to be everything his caretakers told him, was the inevitable response to a chaotic world swirling with a mix of hostility and neglect from multiple sources.

. . .

The enemy is very close.

Sandy M.

Sandy is a violinist who, as a child, had enjoyed a very close relationship with his father, also a musician. When we first met, he had stopped playing altogether, having developed severe symptomatic pain in his neck and shoulder that prevented him from even holding the instrument. He was radically estranged from his parents, resenting his mother who had become 300 pounds and bedridden, commanding all his father's attention. Before his first session, he asked if I would write anything down he wanted to remember, and around the one-hour mark, he declared, "I never knew I loved my parents so much." Such is the power of MDMA to show us how we really feel, who we really are. It never lies.

I had been very depressed since I was a teenager. I'd tried conventional therapy. I'd done some large group awareness trainings. I heard about breathwork; I read Tony Schwartz and his interview with Stan Grof; I don't know. I was desperate, and I really would've tried pretty much anything. I wasn't expecting it to work.

I did some more reading and had an idea of what to expect. I was prepared to just have an amusing story to tell, like this strange thing that I did with a bunch of weirdos at the breathwork group. I sat for another person first, so that was helpful, because I got to see the range of acceptable behaviours in the room. I think that sort of loosened me up to go with whatever I was feeling.

Then, when I did the session, I felt a tingling in my fingers (*tetany*) quite quickly. Then, nothing happened for a while. Toward the end of the session, my head was suddenly suffused with light, and it was as though somebody had poured a pitcher of warm water over my head. I smelled urine, and I had a sudden, very deep, intuitive understanding that everything I'd suffered, it had happened for a reason. It blew me away, because it was an epiphany. It was a real epiphany, and I believed it utterly.

It was a watershed moment in my life and in my emotional, mental well-being. It's hard to describe it any better than that.

The most depressing thing about depression is the idea that, for me, I was suffering needlessly. There was no point to my suffering. I guess the corollary to that is what sort of higher power would allow me to suffer without any reason? Which in turn, made me more depressed.

The epiphany totally turned that around. I realised that everything I had gone through, my abusive childhood, sexual traumas, depression itself, all those things had meaning and contributed to who I was and would have value for myself and others. I probably had read that prior to doing it, but I had never really felt it, and certainly not on that deep a level.

I don't know how many other epiphanies like that I've had in my life. It ranks on the same level as seeing my dad in tears after my mom passed away and realising how much he loved her. I had no idea how much he loved her; and it's lasted. I was not cured of depression overnight. I still have wrestled with ups and downs, but I have never been close to killing myself since that experience. I have never really seriously considered giving up. No matter what the circumstance is now, I feel like there has to be meaning in it.

Part of the solution is in the process of finding meaning and not just taking a combative stance toward something, not attacking my depression with interventions and medications and whatnot, and finding meaning in that suffering and the suffering that we are enduring presently, with climate change and all these things. There is meaning in all of it, and to me, that's faith.

That experience gave me faith. It made my love of God self-evident. I never knew I loved God so much. I never knew I loved my parents so much.

It just became so apparent to me, that my view of God was mostly about my view of my parents, this idea that God was absent, not really concerned about my welfare and whatnot. These are negative feelings that I brought with me from some of the ways in which I was raised. It became clear that the only thing standing between me and loving God was my own baggage. It had nothing to do with God.

All the doubts and the resentments and whatnot were suddenly irrelevant.

I had a number of MDMA sessions. It seems like so long ago. I had an experience where my heart opened. I suddenly realised how much I had hurt my mother, as much as she had hurt me. Part of my origin story is that I am the helpless victim of her psychotic episodes. She was very loving, but she was also very mentally ill. I recognised that I had a part in that, and I wrote her a love letter. I'm so grateful that I had that experience before she died, because I had a few conversations with her that were connected from the heart in a way that I thought was totally gone.

The last session I did had sort of a delayed effect. I remember the next day, or a couple of days later, I was walking home, and I suddenly was overwhelmed. This was another epiphany. I was overwhelmed with how selfish I was, just how much my own regard for myself had informed my entire sense of being.

I sensed that I was enormously selfish at my core and far more so than I had ever realised. I started crying. I had a bit of a freak-out. Not long after that, I ended up going to my first AA meeting. It's been four and a half years since I've had a drink or any kind of substance, and that's been an interesting, completely unexpected twist in this journey, because it started off very much involved in those things. I had no sense of the extent to which I also used substances to check out of my daily life.

Even while doing this medicine work, I would stop drinking for about a month or two after each session, but my routine was to come home from work and have a giant bottle of red wine, and drink and smoke myself into a stupor, watching TV every night, which is hard to believe, considering how I spend my time now. That's how I coped with my depression. It's one of the many things that I tried. I remember my sister calling me once, very depressed, and I said, "Well, have you tried getting high?" That was my antidepressant.

I did also start having experiences in my dream life that were very psychedelic, profound, and amazing. For example, I started having many lucid dreams and out-of-body experiences. When I stopped drinking, I thought, "Well, this is great. I figured it out. I found the loophole. I don't need anybody else. I can just go to sleep every night and blast off." I had some amazing experiences, like I met my deceased mother, and I had a talk with her in a lucid dream.

She was just the most perfect version of herself that could be possible. If you strip away all the baggage of mental illness, this is who she was at her core. She was talking to me, and I was just amazed that this was happening, and I was writing down what she said. The only thing I remembered when I woke up was she told me to stay in the rooms, which is AA slang for continuing to go to meetings and stick with the programme.

I had several experiences like that, that were just very moving. Then, I started to have some darker experiences, experiences of being harassed and persecuted by nasty figures.

So, I contacted a number of people. One was Scott Sparrow, who's a psychologist in Texas and author of the first book on lucid dreaming published in the West. We did a phone therapy thing for a while, and he was terrific. He had a very balanced view of the whole thing. He talked about these compensatory shadow experiences, which go hand in hand with an accelerated path of development, so being involved in a slow path and a quick path, and the quick path, which I think involves states like this, induced through various means, is radically transformative and can also be very scary. I got to the point where I felt like it was not good for my emotional well-being to go any further.

I looked high and low for some kind of system of support that felt wholesome, but it was difficult to find, because I had many experiences of learning a little bit more about a group, or a person, or somebody holding themselves up as a spiritual teacher, and finding that their work was very much compromised by their ego. For the record, I never felt that with my attendant; I always felt so taken care of.

I feel like right now, I'm being called to deepen my engagement in worldly affairs, and there's a part of me that still longs for this other work. I walked in that MDMA treatment room with the beautiful ceiling and the turtle poster, and I think about how present I was to love on that couch, and I think about how difficult it is for me, sometimes, to access that.

The closest I get, and it's pretty close, is when I'm rigorously honest with my girlfriend, when I'm very, very painfully honest with her. It's a type of intimacy that I have never experienced before. It's a meeting of peers, soul-mates. We speak the same language.

I also have a friend who started an organisation with Ram Dass called Human Kindness Foundation. Her husband taught meditation and yoga to inmates, and she set up his literature and managed the nonprofit. Her entire spiritual practice was built around service. She meditated her entire life. I told her about some of these experiences, and she was curious about it.

But what I found was that my ego got very wrapped up in feeling like some sort of guru. This guy in Texas told me that my experiences, or my facility or abilities in that arena were uncommon. I very quickly decided that I was going to put together a website and promote myself as a teacher. Very quickly, my ego stepped in, and I puffed myself up. It took me a few months to see it happening, but right before I pushed Go on this whole plan, I just couldn't do it. I just could not ignore the reality of what was happening, which was that I was trying to make a buck, get some notoriety, and some respect.

The enemy is very close.

We need to have the ability to respond, our response-ability, to whatever it is we carry. Sadly, much of the time we may be ignorant of what we are dealing with and what we truly feel, so how can we respond meaningfully when we are confused about what it is we are responding to? By opening himself to a wider view with breathwork and subsequently MDMA, Sandy was able to understand emotionally and cognitively how much he loved his parents. This enabled the resumption of their relationship, engagement with Alcoholics Anonymous, a tender personal relationship, and a worldview that informs his work as a schoolteacher.

Sandy's testimony speaks to the power of his honesty; to experience and acknowledge the love he truly felt for his parents and for God, and to be open to insights and epiphanies occurring during and after the medicine sessions. Once we are opened to the truth of the matter, that truth can no longer be denied and will continue with insistence and at every opportunity, to press upon our psyches by releasing to us whatever it can, partial or whole, from the trauma it has captured. Dreams, and especially lucid dreams, are very close cousins to the medicine work. In both forms, we reveal ourselves to ourselves and in lucid dreaming we experience ordinary consciousness and non-ordinary consciousness simultaneously for an extended period. This dual awareness is an extraordinary and fruitful stance within which we can experience more than one aspect of ourselves at the same time. The honesty this individual employs in facing his shortcomings also pierces his schemes for enrichment, notoriety and respect, foiling an incipient guru-grandiosity trip. The medicine itself does not lie, and if we are true to ourselves in every moment while under its influence, neither can we.

• • •

It is not a verbal experience.

Amadeus.

Once the terrible darkness with which Amadeus had lived met with MDMA, it began to dissolve. His father was a businessman and a talented musician, whose relationship with his firstborn ran the gamut of rare affection to extreme violence; he was, by turns, a sensitive, accomplished cellist and a violent man with erratic mood swings. Their relationship might have resolved over time had not his father died in a plane crash when Amadeus was fifteen years old, an event that he has subsequently learned was a deliberate act of sabotage by the Soviet Union during the Cold War.

Amadeus's emotional development was stalled at the height of this loss, and he carried the complexity of unresolved feelings forward into his life. Upon his father's death, he became the head of a traumatised family, comprising his mother, brother, and sister, an honoured responsibility he carried forward as phobia and fear. Some work with psychedelics had amplified these to a point where he became overwhelmed, but the sweet feelings of ease precipitated by MDMA was exactly the corrective this traumatised individual needed.

Before trying MDMA, I had conventional therapy in Europe for about a year, a year and a half, which could have been more hindering and destructive if I had stayed longer. It certainly didn't help. It wasn't bad, but it didn't help. I had another eight months in Hamburg, and that didn't help that much either. I did some one-on-one therapy, a combination of primal and Gestalt. It gave me a certain amount of release. I went once a week or something like that. Then, I met a traditional psychoanalyst who works like (child development psychologist) D. W. Winnicott, a really good guy. About eight months into it, I couldn't afford him any longer.

My wife and I had marriage problems, and we went to somebody he referred us to; then, the decision came that we would separate. Subsequently, the woman who was our marriage counsellor became my therapist. I'd been reading Stanislav Grof looking for answers. One day, I looked at my therapist, and she looked like she could be my mother. I thought to myself, here I am at the age of thirty-eight boo-hooing about how difficult life is, in the presence of a woman who could be my mother, and I said, "This is just not right. This can't go on like this." I told her, and I think she was shocked, but I really liked her a lot. She was absolutely a wonderful human being.

Then, I got involved with breathwork groups, once or twice a year. I also had a few psychedelic sessions where somebody I trusted sat with me; I wouldn't want to have missed them, but it was more like an exploration than anything else.

By this point, I was about to give up, because I wasn't getting out of my misery.

One summer day, I had my first MDMA experience, and it was

a revelation. What shocked me the most, in a good way, was realising the amount of fear that I was walking around with all the time, and that it was right underneath the surface. Through working with MDMA for about six years, on average about three sessions a year, slowly and gradually certain things started to soften and symptoms started to disappear.

The first eight to ten medicine sessions were just amazing, because every time something seemed to be finished, I seemed to discover something else. For the first one, I lay there on this couch, and I was sweating profusely like I was in a sauna. I had a smile on my face, and I realised, my God, I've been walking around with this fear all my life, understandably so from the kind of experiences that I had as a child.

That perspective, the ability to look at myself, even if it's just for a few hours and a few days—although the first one lasted for about two or three months for me—is incredibly helpful. The attendant who sat with me said, "This is who you really are." I'm thinking, "This is who I really am? That sweet guy?" The peaceful feeling stayed with me. It's changed my life, and it saved my life.

I would never, ever use MDMA as a crutch or go to it as an escape hatch, just to not have to deal with the inevitable slings and arrows of outrageous fortune. I'm not a medical or psychiatric professional, but I believe from what I know and understand that this work is ideal for people who are profoundly traumatised. It's a way to get to the underlying issue in a gentle, relatively fast way.

The MDMA experience goes very, very deep, because it is nonverbal. One of the things that happened to me was that my muscles started to vibrate and twitch with muscle fasciculation, like plucking the string on a musical instrument. That's the amount of tension that was there. That has decreased enormously.

That's what MDMA does. You're inevitably confronted with the feeling, how you feel physically and emotionally. It's not a verbal experience. You're not trying to explain something. You're finding the release.

That first session was such a revelation, and it brought such a smile to my face. I couldn't believe that this is who I am, and that all this fear that I had walked around with kept me always on guard. I'm a lot less on guard now; even my fear of large dogs has started to disappear. Also, my fear of heights has diminished. Other symptoms have either totally diminished or decreased significantly. I would say there isn't a single symptom that hasn't decreased by at least 50 percent.

Through being reconnected to his feelings of survivor guilt and extreme emotional grief, Amadeus could come to terms with the loss of his father, an event that had precluded any possibility of resolution of their extremely difficult relationship. He could gain some measure of closure of this family trauma, to reestablish coherence with his family, to be attentive and present for his mother at her passing and to fulfil his role as head of the family with careful administration of their shared estate. Despite his love, passion and respect for classical music, he has been unable to work as a musician for much of his life, only now becoming able to consider performing again. The loss of any ability to pursue our career is huge, undermining confidence in our God-given talents and leading to ever-greater feelings of helplessness.

• • •

So much to express, it is almost inexpressible.

Ludwig P.

Anger is a reactive emotion; we feel angry as the result of some slight or hurt, and for some, it is the only feeling they know. Anger has been pathologised as unseemly, and we are at pains to control it in our lives as the results may be not to our, or our fellows, liking. But if we can understand the extent of the abuse and neglect that was visited upon us by whomever, but particularly our parents, then the expression of anger becomes righteous. Context is the thing; we need to allow ourselves to become angry in a safe and supported setting, expressing feelings that have been inexpressible, up to and including murderous feelings. This experiential contact with how we really feel, and the full-bodied expression of same in a safe and supported environment, absent societal controls, is key. It's the niceness that kills us.

Before starting the medicine work, my life was disjointed with little holding me together. I fully believed in the past, and it was ruling my life. I had very little control of things. Although I had been working in psychotherapy for many years, and it was very beneficial in terms of identifying the causes and issues and mitigating the symptoms, I had not gotten to the core feelings. What was I feeling? I knew I was angry. Every step I took during the day came with a jolt of anger, for example, someone blocking my way in the train, a surly sounding voice taking my food order to deliver, the way my doorman greeted me, a man who frowned at my dog—I took it all personally, and it cut deeply, making me want to kill the world. The two main ways I took it out on myself, or got relief, whichever side of the coin you pick, was heavy drugs and anonymous sex. I was unable to connect in the world any other way.

Then, my therapist suggested the possibility of work with MDMA. I was excited, almost thrilled about the prospect of a way to get to the bottom of it, finally! I would break through and be free; this is what I hoped for desperately. I met my attendant for the consultation, and he gave me hope. That was the beginning.

I trusted him right away. He was interested in me and in helping me. I trusted the surroundings. It felt good. He even had a dog, which closed the deal for me. I have always said that dogs are the best people. I have seen both my dogs go crazy chasing after deer, turn on each other in the heat of the hunt, and a few moments later (after I broke them up) they are best friends again; what a way to live life! In any case, my attendant explained the medicine to me. I had taken quite a bit of MDMA in the past, recreationally, and even then, I thought of it as medicine, even though I never fully formulated that thought. Medicine, because it makes you feel better, it opens you up, so that you can face what's inside without the fear, judgement, ridicule, hatred, anxiety, and so on. I had a handful of sessions over more than a year and chipped away at memories, ideas, concepts…and I think all of this was necessary to get to the point where I could have my breakthrough session. In the previous sentence, I had actually put quotation marks around breakthrough, then I deleted them. Need I say more? Probably.

I turned fifty this year in May. I had about sixty people up to my house in the countryside. It was a love fest with people from all stages of my life in one place. I *felt* good.

And by early afternoon the next day, they were gone. I was ALONE, all caps, screaming, devastating loneliness ripping at my heart, tearing my limbs off and leaving me a bloody stumpy mess on the floor. What the fuck? To stop this immediately, I scooped up five or six Klonopin and passed out. From that point until mid-July, I swirled deeper and deeper into a death spiral, sinking into self-loathing, pity, angry at the world, all accentuated by a recurrence of regular drug use, anonymous sex, and danger. I was regressing to my habits before therapy. There were moments where I believed that I would be electrocuted if I switched on a light, or that I was going to have a stroke or heart attack, because my heart felt like it was heaving through my chest. At one point, I even drove myself to a clinic where they kept me for a while to see if my blood pressure would abate. My head was out to get me. I was devastated; fifty and utterly ALONE.

In mid-July, I committed to a goal of no "bad" behaviour until my session, which was scheduled for a month later. I stuck to that. My prior sessions had given me the foundation of hope I needed, and I felt—not thought—that this time something HAD to shift. That feeling was spot on, and as it turned out in synch with the direction my attendant gave me at the outset of the session—feel, don't think. See the feeling for what it is, in the bright, unadulterated light of the medicine. Let the medicine work. And so, I did.

First, I allowed myself to just feel good. I let the medicine wash over me like a wave of feathers, trusting and embracing it. When I began to follow and articulate my thoughts, I was provided with gentle, internal direction to feel what was going on at that moment. And after about an hour of allowing the medicine to work, I saw it: A baby crying hysterically in a completely lightless room. Terror! I knew that the baby had been abandoned for days and was starving and terrified in the pitch-black room. And in that moment, I realised that I had spent my entire adulthood defensive and angry to avoid feeling that fear, the gaping gnaws of pain and hurt of an abandoned starving baby.

After this session, I sensed something had lifted—the veil of shame and secrecy I lived with. The hardwired fear from so long ago lost its hold, but not easily. I spent a full two weeks after the session on vacation (luckily) at my country house, and the first night I had a graphic dream. The fear was not going to give up easily. Here is an excerpt of the e-mail I wrote to my attendant two days after the session.

> "Dreamt my mother was carrying a live baby around in a plastic container with a lid, AND she was pregnant, so I pushed her down on the street at a bus stop, and a bus came by at that minute. I waved for the bus driver to stop, but I don't think frantically, and he went straight ahead with one wheel rolling over my mother who was prone on the street. Instead of crushing her, the bus just rolled over her, like she wasn't a mass of fluids and bone. At the end, I woke, wondering if it had killed her and the unborn baby."

After that, I had insomnia for almost all of the remaining two weeks. I emailed my attendant frequently about my experiences during those two weeks. Here are excerpts:

August 25th

I often forget that I am not truly alone and wake up terrified. I am noticing the way I behave by myself and with people. All of this is hard and stressful. I feel like there is something inside me that is sick and dying, and I'm sad a lot, and it's hard being alone and dealing with all this, but I know I am not alone.

August 27th

Hadn't really slept for a few days until last night. Last night, just as I was about to doze off shortly after my head hit the pillow, I was jolted awake by a vision of pure white static electricity and lightning and a sound like a sonic boom, lasting less than a second. I realised, then, that my mind was fighting hard to keep the past in control. I didn't fall asleep until a few hours later, when I finally realised I didn't have to be angry, because I wasn't falling asleep, and I could take care of myself and give myself advice—breathe in, breathe out; calm.

August 28th

It was back to no sleep last night. This lack of sleep is fraying my nerves. Maybe I am afraid of the panic that will set upon me when I open my eyes in the morning. I noticed I was wired, tense and angry before sleep last night and I didn't judge it. But I can't keep not sleeping, being afraid to go to bed, tossing and turning, looking at my clock one minute and it is 12:00 p.m., then again, it is 1:00 a.m., etc. I need to resolve the sleep disorder myself, to dream, to have flashing, lightning, electric images—my panic image of electricity and electrifying myself, dying.

To this last bit, my attendant responded:

Always remember that the worst is already over, long gone, and that by evoking such feelings, we are evoking traces of past wounds and false ideas that we still carry from not knowing how to un-carry. The work you have done has loosened the bonds that bind these issues to you as if they were the truth of you; they are not, and with your conscious consideration can be seen as the falsehoods they really are.

Thanks to my resolve, based on what I had awoken to at the session—the realisation that I am no longer alone, dying in a lightless room—and with my attendant's assistance (his compassion and wisdom reached out from my iPhone during those subsequent two weeks), I am HERE to tell the story.

It is important to me to tell you how I am doing. At the time of writing this, it has been about six weeks since the breakthrough session, and about twelve weeks since I stopped using any kind of destructive substance or engaging in any kind of destructive activity. I am back to my routine of weekdays in the city and weekends in the country, and the city has presented its myriad of challenges, but I am seeing things anew and clearly. I am happy and confident a lot more of the time. Am I still afraid? Sure. Is there untangling still to be done? Of course! The screams of that baby should not be stifled, but they can be soothed and softened. Fear was only there to protect me, and so when it shows up now, I acknowledge it, but I go on with my day (I envision it sits on my right shoulder, like a miniature leprechaun, but I am not compelled to listen to it. I have the right to decide in what measure I will take its advice, if at all). I will leave you with an excerpt from a recent e-mail to my attendant.

Sept 22nd

"Things are much better. Day by day without judging. It's nice. Life is easier. So much to express, it is almost inexpressible. I feel good finally. I can meet the world."

● ● ●

We need to know the truth, the whole truth and nothing but the truth about what occurred during our upbringing to make sense of the self-destructive behaviours that have resulted from it. We may know intellectually that anonymous sex leaves us feeling disgusted, and that heavy drugs, from both the street or the pharmacy, can damage us, but we are helpless to control our desire to use and abuse. The truth, however, sets us free to understand the very source of the fear we are trying to self-medicate away, and by so doing diminishes its power to affect our behaviour. Once the unknown becomes known to us, we claim our own agency and can become better able to interpret our feelings as they arise and to act upon them appropriately.

FINAL TESTIMONY

Beyond Trauma

"Those who love truth must investigate many things."

HERACLITUS

The preceding testimonies are from individuals who presented
with the symptoms of trauma and PTSD as expressed in their
testimonies (A. Z., who gratefully noted the absence of trauma
in his life, was the exception that proved the rule as, arguably,
were the couple, S. C. and J. C., who had come to work on the
challenge of blending their two families following their divorces
in midlife).

The trauma responsible for their dysfunctional symptoms, up to
and including PTSD, were captured and held 'incohate' within
them per Ivor Browne's hypothesis of Unexperienced Experience.
This condition was adequately understood by Freud's colleague
Charcot in his book 'Psychological Healing' published in the 1860s,
which he references as follows: "All the patients seem to have
had the evolution of their lives checked; they are 'attached' upon
an object that they cannot get beyond." Through the action of

MDMA to flood the brain with serotonin, creating the essential feeling of safety, the psyches of these clients had found the trauma, or 'object' per Charcot's rendering, and had become unattached from it following the psyche's release.

However, the known effect of MDMA is to produce feelings of ecstasy in the user, and it is interesting to see how this ability plays out in a client who, having previously worked with somatic experiencing and other means, had processed a lot of her trauma. She therefore has no major trauma within her as she enters the session. This testimony is included to convey the power of the medicine as it opens us to the boundlessness and profound mystery of our psyche. This includes expansive visions, entities and experiences of past lives far beyond the limited purview of orthodox psychiatry or psychology, the focus of which is upon the amelioration of symptoms of fear, depression, and anxiety, not upon the underlying cause or causes of these symptoms. These symptoms are then classified with such names as OCD, Bipolar Disorder, Schizoaffective Disorder and so on that are detailed in the 'bible' of their profession, the Diagnostic and Statistical Manual (DSM), currently in its Fifth Edition.

From the point of view of the medicine's healing potential, it is interesting to note how, once exposed to MDMA, this client's attention becomes bifurcated. She references things in the here-and-now of ordinary consciousness, the music, the blanket, the attendant, while simultaneously expressing what she is experiencing within herself in non-ordinary, even transpersonal, consciousness; pain, Africa, beauty, and so on. In a person with trauma and PTSD symptoms, this is exactly the condition the psyche needs to understand that the terrible emotional memory it captured and has been carrying for years no longer exists, that the individual is now listening to sweet music under a beloved blanket, that it is not 1992 anymore, and all is now well. Once it can experientially understand that was then and this is now, it realises the emergency is past and releases the captured traumatic memory as swiftly as it captured it in the first instance. This is the action of Unexperienced Experience expressed in so many testimonies, but in this instance, we see the action of the medicine when it does not encounter 'an object' per Charcot, the traumatic memory, and is simply able to freely expand to the furthest reaches of consciousness.

• • •

I'm in different dimensions all the time. I'm here and flying around. Different lives.

L. A. S.

The following lines were spoken by L. A. S., a South African clinical psychologist who works with trauma victims in London, during her first exploratory session. Presented here as single lines, each were spoken by her to the attendant while she was exposed to the medicine and were written down verbatim. We see her becoming relaxed within minutes of taking the first dose, and soon thereafter, she was fully engaged within the transpersonal realm for the remainder of her time on the couch.

The following notes were taken over the first three hours of her six-hour session, and each line represents a discrete statement made by her after returning to silence. The interval between statements varied between a few minutes and a few moments. The session continued in this vein until its conclusion, and following these notes spoken from within the session itself, L. A. S. writes post-session of her experience.

I am aware of a lot of anxiety.

Little more relaxed with tingling all over my arms.

Seeing so much pain in the human condition. It's not my pain.

The immensity of it. All transpersonal. Become a conduit.

My heart feels so big.

It's all transpersonal but I feel very
grounded here on the couch.

Pain. Suffering. Is it showing me many
different lives I have had?

Archetypes.

Music is so beautiful.

Showing me the ravages of trauma.

In the midst of this I feel very peaceful.

How does one transmute all the pain?

I feel so grateful.

It's darkness. (sighs)

I can feel so much love.

Ribbons of light in the darkness.

Still doesn't feel personal.

I see my life. So much love for me. (hands on heart)

So beautiful.

Many images in India.

A shrine.

Animals.

I can hold everything.

In Africa.

Pain. So much beauty.

Love.

So beautiful.

Such good music.

British flag.

My heart is so open.

There is certainly not anything to be afraid of.
Some jungles, animals going in and out of trees.
My heart is so big.
It's amazing.
I can't believe I've never done this before. It's so magnificent.
I think this is the way out of all the darkness.
Oh, my goodness!
It feels so beautiful.
Love does change everything.
Love is the only thing that matters.
I think this is one of the best things I have ever done in my life.
It's really holy.
Conduit is the only word for what I am.
This music!
Just basking in love.
So beautiful.
I'm totally aware of my body. I haven't left my body at all.
The music; little rabbits bouncing.
The music is like exclamation points.
I just want to lie here forever.
I feel ecstatic.
I think this is the way to transmute all that sadness into light.
Thank you. For what you do, not just for me.
I feel the capacity for us humans to have such huge hearts.
There is nothing to be afraid of.
I think this is the way to transmute the pain
and trauma in the world. So interesting.
Now I just feel good and relaxed. Here in the beauty.
People don't know their hearts are so big. A
woman, the archetype of ugliness. In the
midst of all the beauty I am seeing.
Holy! Holy! Holy!

Thanks for being so present.

I'm totally conscious now.

Part of me is weeping for all that I've

learned. Not just me weeping.

Weeping with gratitude.

An African woman dipping her toe into water. Flamingoes.

She has something on her head.

I just love this blanket that's covering me.

It's a gift I'm giving myself, to close my

eyes and see all these people.

I've travelled the globe today, India, Africa, all over.

I want everyone I know to do this.

I'm seeing all these images, all my past lives.

The whole gamut of human emotions.

I'm witnessing the whole spectrum, all its beauty, all its fear.

Children in Africa, laughing, smiling.

Some of your grief is being transmuted right now. Now I'm

holding it. Tears and tears and tears. Darkness in my abdomen.

Some people crying inside my heart. Africa, in my heart.

I feel so grounded, so here, and I can

choose to share this or not.

A baby squirrel being murdered.

I feel I am holding everything in my

heart. Russia, China. Ukraine.

So much pain in the elephant kingdom.

I'm a conduit I think. I chose this role.

Those were all my past lives, millions

of them. Part of my experience.

I feel a gentleness in my soul, a gratitude

in me. I have so much to do.

Music. The evolution of humanity. So much torture, so

much rage, so much beauty. The holocaust. So much love.

Do you feel a lightness in you? I can see it so much.
Transmuting people's darkness to light and love.
On a bigger scale. For mankind, I want to take
it into my arms and transmute all the pain.
There's so much goodness in me and the work of
transmuting their pain. I don't know how to.
Now a very British lady walking by with her handbag.
No reason ever to be anxious.
There's energy streaming, streaming out of my arms
and legs. Light is just coming out of me. My arms.
I just feel ecstasy.
Now I can feel the pain. Heart!
Tears. I picture Atlas with the world on top of him. I
think I have a big role to play in transmuting this pain.
I'm feeling all those pains in my heart.
Violence. The pain in Africa, so much.
Transmuting it for all these people
in Africa. I am a huge mother.
This sadness does not go away. It's in the human body.
I feel I am transmuting. I just don't know how to do
it. My heart is so open I feel pain as well as pleasure.
Mother Theresa is talking to me. (arms out, hands open)
It's not Mother Theresa. Who is that saint? Saint Francis, yes.
All these people are here to help me.
I'm in different dimensions all the time. I'm
here and flying around. Different lives.
Different types of me, faces.
A transgender person with orange lipstick, high
heels. Blond hair, really big breasts.
Shiva-Shakti embrace?
This pain, so weird.
My body, so much pain.

A different universe thanks me for transmuting. Thank you.
Spending a lot of time in Africa, so much pain.
Shaman.
Seeing light green, Egyptian gold chain. Grateful.
I'm so sorry. Killed someone in another life, I've had
so many lives, so much energy transmuted.
Energy running out of me. Feel like a warrior. That's grief.
Old. Old. Old. And not mine.
By myself.
I am an herbalist and gathering herbs in so many past lives.
Seeing a woman totally dancing in the '20s. Black Hair. It's me.
I went through so many lives.
I'm here to transmute all the darkness. (vibrates)
My goodness!

• • •

My decision to partake in MDMA was twofold: First, as a therapist with many clients who have plant medicine experiences, I wanted to experience firsthand what they were going through. And second, I have been actively working on my own healing and growth—somatically, psychologically, and spiritually—via meditation, therapy, and energy work for the last two decades, to keep growing and knowing that I could only take my clients as far as I have gone. My expectation was that MDMA would help me integrate pockets of unprocessed trauma giving me more spaciousness and light in my body and mind.

I sat on the comfortable couch in a panelled room with a maroon carpet, tonnes of books, tribal sculptures, and a little dog scampering around, grounding the energy. The attendant had reassured me that the experience would be exactly what I need. I ingested the first pill, donned eyeshades, and lay down. I felt a little anxious. The attendant had previously explained how Ivor Browne, M.D. felt that returning to unprocessed traumatic experiences in an altered state of consciousness could allow us to gently process trauma.

The MDMA started to take effect. I felt like I was watching a movie of the human condition from the beginning of humanity—such ravages of trauma all depicted by humans—so much sadness, anger, poverty, pain, genocides, including the Holocaust and several in Africa, slavery, trafficking, refugees, addicts, so much of humans' inhumanity to others, including the animals and our earth. I saw a despotic cruel haughty leader, huddled masses, skeletons, greed. And they were all me in past lives. I was killed and a killer, a giver, and a receiver of pain; I was greedy and a sufferer of poverty and hunger. I was powerful and part of the masses. And the pain and fear I felt inside me was profound. Interspersed and following were images containing much beauty, goodness, simplicity—people laughing, giving, dancing, creating, discovering, eating, loving, sharing, giving, and taking of plants and herbs as friends and with friends. So many thousands of past lives, some predominated by pain, some predominated by pleasure, and one image/expression acted as a microcosm of the entire life. Human images appeared from all over the world—Africa, India, China, Ukraine, Yugoslavia, England, Greece engaged in different ways of being human. And then, I saw Avalakotishvara with 108 arms to give kindness, St. Francis (was that me or is he talking to me?), archetypes/goddesses of the feminine, the mother and her gentle power washing the earth, and I was one with all these images. My heart was opening to hold all the pain as well as all the beauty.

And then, all the books I have ever read, and many I have not, passed by me, seemingly talking to me and teaching me—the first bound books from Gutenberg's printing press, Greek literature, Shakespeare, spiritual texts from all religions, and on and on, contemporary books on psychology, spirituality, philosophy, systems, constellations, anthropology, consciousness—I could see it all, feel it all and felt grateful for the knowledge and wisdom. Classical and contemporary art and architectural beauty, in all their forms, all passing by me to reflect their gifts of beauty and have the opportunity for gratitude to those of us who brought these great works through. Oh, much wonder. We are acting as conduits for all this beauty,

An image of a tall African woman, smiling at me across the continents, reminding me that we are one, and that I am she, and she is me. Is she a past life, a parallel life, intuitive guidance that I must visit or work in Africa? I felt like Mother Earth holding us all—the pain, beauty, wonder, exquisiteness of it all. Just as I was feeling like I was holding humanity, I saw a rabbit scurrying across a detonated land area and she was absorbing some of the pain of the human condition. I saw hunters kill animals for joy. I felt the sadness and wisdom of the elephants at our cruelty and greed. I could, again, feel and see the pain in the world for humans, for animals and for our Mother Earth. I could feel the transgenerational and collective nature of these traumas and knew, if we as a species want to grow and evolve, we need to transmute all this trauma, and I need to act as a conduit to transmute some of this. My whole body was vibrating for hours trying to release some of the pain in the world.

I didn't know if I had no boundaries, or if the world was within me, or if I was tapping into the unified whole or akashic field.

I was astounded at the beauty and holiness of every moment. Holy, holy, holy—kadosh, kadosh, kadosh! Julian Bream was playing, and I was trying to tap into his life, and how he channelled this lovely music. Everything felt holy and shimmering with fragile beauty.

Then, I saw myself in a different dimension—I was whiteness and light and not human but definitely me. I was such pure goodness and gentleness. When I looked at humans from this dimension, I saw they had different degrees of light and different colours of energy ribbons in their energy bodies. In this other dimension, I was learning how to do energy work to transmute others' pain, to simply remove it from their experience. I saw someone afflicted with such intense grief and desperation in Africa, and I was able to transmute and remove his pain and change the lens in which he saw his life. I was really proud of myself and went to my counsel, who were my teachers, much more experienced than I was. I had one main teacher, and there were another five or so in the group. They felt very wise and very kind and felt so experienced that I felt so honoured they were my teachers. Meanwhile, my heart was stretching and opening wider, so wide and expanded, it hurt a little. I was told that this is my purpose—to transmute pain on earth as well, and that my therapy practice is only part of it. I asked if I could transmute the pain of my husband, my children, and was told that I could do it a little, but that, ultimately, it is their journey. I need to keep learning about energy and receiving all I am given. As I saw all these divine mothers passing by, I realised that my life purpose is to mother as much of the earth, the people, and the animals that I can. I felt sad that my parents were unable to see me as I was growing up, because they were unable to see my gentle goodness as it did not really attune with them. I felt such deep love for my children. I saw myself dying in this life, and it was a lovely ending.

Since the session, I no longer have any anxiety, fear, or sadness—the medicine transmuted all the pain and fear I had, even though I was unaware that I carried it. There is no longer negative self-judgement or blame. I can feel my uniqueness and beauty and purpose, and I know all this happened in my every cell, and I will never experience it again.

I keep wanting to put this into an intellectual framework and structure, but part of me is realising that it doesn't matter if I saw many of my own past lives and growth or humanity's evolution. It doesn't matter if the smile from the African woman near the Limpopo River in Africa is a past/parallel life or guidance to tell me to visit/work in Africa. It doesn't matter if I am feeling another's pain in my body that needs to be released, or if I am learning to transmute my own. It doesn't matter if my parents didn't recognise my unique loveliness when I was little; I chose it, so I could recognise it myself now. Everything that happens, I now know, is for our own growth and evolution, and we, or our guides, plant this for our benefit. Without a doubt, I can feel our oneness and our unity. To say I feel grateful to the attendant for this experience is an enormous understatement.

* * *

Further Acknowledgements

The attendants to the work presented in this book offer their deepest respect to the giants of trauma recovery upon whose shoulders we stand. For these individuals, trauma has been their life-work, often precipitated by their own traumatic experiences; on this point, at least, we may claim fraternity. Many such clinicians and researchers have dedicated themselves to work therapeutically with trauma victims while simultaneously seeking to find the common threads to the conundrum of trauma that has confounded clinicians and patients since time immemorial.

We gratefully acknowledge the work of the following pioneers, whose work with trauma has informed our work with the medicine by clearly identifying the body as the repository of trauma.

John E. Mack, M.D., whose Pulitzer Prizewinning book, *A Prince of our Disorder* examined the life of T. E. Lawrence (of Arabia), practised and taught at Harvard Medical School until his untimely death in 2004. His professional focus was on the effects of trauma upon the individual, but in the public sphere he co-founded the Center for Psychology and Social Change (CPSC) in 1989. CPSC engaged with political and social institutions, including the UN, to examine the underlying psychological reasons for war. Dr. Mack's mentorship affirmed and supported our own work in practising the healing potential of non-ordinary consciousness.

Ivor Browne, M.D., whose 1990 paper, "Psychological Trauma, or Unexperienced Experience" informs our work in ways beyond calculation. This article states, "Simply, when something happens to us we do not experience all of it at once," and observations from this practice affirm the truth of this hypothesis. Browne's career was focused on improving the conditions of mental care in Ireland, and he conceived and was the director of The Irish Foundation for Human Development. He was particularly engaged with efforts to move away from the 'warehousing' of patients in hospitals by pivoting toward establishing effective community centers to treat individuals in need.

Bessel van der Kolk, M.D., has focused his psychiatric lens on the neuro-biological underpinnings of PTSD for over forty years, becoming a leading spokesman for the understanding that the body is the repository of traumatic memories. This is reflected in his seminal book, *The Body Keeps the Score*, which has informed our behaviour and practice. Dr. van der Kolk continues to refine his groundbreaking work as Medical Director at the Trauma Center at JRI in Brookline, Massachusetts, publishing extensively on the impact of trauma on cognitive development in children and adults, disassociation, the psychobiology of trauma and other related topics. Dr. van der Kolk's current research examines how trauma affects memory processes, including brain imaging studies of PTSD victims.

Peter Levine, Ph.D., studied medical biophysics and was introduced to mind-body techniques at the Esalen Institute in Big

Sur, California during the 1960s. During his studies, he had been introduced to the phenomenon of tonic immobility, a condition expressed by animals for over 500 million years. Animals, when frightened and unable to employ either fight-or-flight, spontaneously enter a non-ordinary state of consciousness and freeze. Building upon this insight over his working life, Dr. Levine developed 'somatic experiencing' (SE), a powerful and effective method of gradual trauma release described in *Waking the Tiger* and other books. SE is taught and practised worldwide.

Each of these trauma specialists acknowledges the essential role of non-ordinary consciousness in the release of traumatic memories.

In this regard, special acknowledgement and sincere gratitude must be made to Michael Mithoefer, M.D. and his wife Annie Mithoefer, B.S.N. and colleagues for their brilliant empirical studies demonstrating MDMA's healing potential. At this writing, Phase I and Phase II trials have been successfully concluded, and their research work will continue until the completion of a Phase III trial involving 200 subjects. The fortitude and persistence required by these indefatigable researchers in pressing the regulatory authorities in the United States to oversee these skillfully designed and successfully executed studies has resulted in a radical extension of our understanding of MDMA's healing potential.

Above all, we honour the clients who have courageously come to work with us after many years living lives of quiet desperation, and who have openheartedly shared their experiences in this book. They wish to bear witness to the releases they have achieved in order that others might benefit from understanding what they, gratefully, have come to understand. It is within those testimonies that the most meaningful information about this medicine work is to be found, shared by the unique voices of people astonished by the gentle power of this medicine. It is our hope that when read in aggregate, they may give the reader a coherent view of the how and why of MDMA work.

These testimonies are offered as contemporaneous examples of trauma release made possible through the responsible use of MDMA. Perhaps, they may contribute to a fuller appreciation of the body's ability to capture and release trauma than currently exists. It is further hoped they may comport with the sentiment expressed by trauma specialist Judith Lewis Herman, M.D., in her highly praised book, *Trauma and Recovery*, that:

> *"Comparison of new treatment methods developed independently by creative pioneers may yield some insight into the underlying common principles."*

From our repeated observations, we respectfully suggest that these outcomes fundamentally serve to demonstrate the truth about the body's intrinsic ability to heal itself. This action, seen in so many of the testimonies, underscores a 1948 statement by Wilhelm Reich, M. D. in which he urges us to consider "the biological basis of the emotional life of man."

Recommended Reading

Browne, Ivor. 2009. *Music and Madness*. Cork: Cork University Press.

Van der Kolk, Bessel A. 2015. *The Body Keeps the Score: Brain, Mind and Body in the Healing of Trauma*. New York: Penguin.

Levine, Peter. 1997. *Waking the Tiger: Healing Trauma: The Innate Capacity to Transform Overwhelming Experiences*. Berkeley, Calif.: North Atlantic Books.

Holland, Julie. 2001. *Ecstasy: The Complete Guide: A Comprehensive Look at the Risks and Benefits of MDMA*. Rochester, Vt.: Park Street Press.

FURTHER READING

Almaas, A. H. 1998. *Facets of Unity; The Enneagram of Holy Ideas*. Berkeley, Diamond Books.

Barber, Charles. 2009. *Comfortably Numb: How Psychiatry is Medicating a Nation*. New York: Vintage Books.

Breuer, Josef and Sigmund Freud. 2012. *Studies on Hysteria*. Lexington: Forgotten Books.

Farber, Seth. 2012. *The Spiritual Gift of Madness: The Failure of Psychiatry and the Rise of the Mad Pride Movement*. Rochester, Vt.: Inner Traditions.

Grof, Stanislav and Hal Zina Bennett. 1993. *The Holotropic Mind: The Three Levels of Human Consciousness and How They Shape Our Lives*. Harper Collins.

Heller, Lawrence and Aline LaPierre. 2012. *Healing Developmental Trauma. How Early Trauma Affects Self-Regulation, Self-Image and the Capacity for Relationship*. Berkeley, Calif.: North Atlantic Books.

Howell, Marilyn. 2011. *Honor Thy Daughter*. Santa Cruz, Calif: Multidisciplinary Association for Psychedelic Studies (MAPS).

Jalom, Irving. 2012. *When Nietzche Wept*. Books On Demand.

Janov, Arthur. 2007. *The Primal Scream: Primal Therapy, the Cure for Neurosis*. Whitefish, Mont: Kessinger.

Jensen, Derrick. 2008. *A Language Older than Words*. Lane Cove, N.S.W.: Finch Publishing.

Jung, Carl. 2013. *Memories, Dreams, Reflections*. Important Books.

Kabat-Zinn, John. 1994. *Wherever You Go, There You Are: Mindfulness Meditation in Everyday Life*. New York: Hyperion.

Kornfield, Jack. 2000. *After the Ecstasy, the Laundry; How the Heart Grows Wise on the Spiritual Path*. Bantam Books.

Leboyer, Frédérick. 1975. *Birth Without Violence*. New York: Knopf.

Laing, R. D. and A. Esterson. 2017. *Sanity, Madness, and the Family*. New York: Routledge.

Lowen, Alexander. 1994. *Bioenergetics*. New York: Penguin/Arkana.

Mack, John E. 1976. *A Prince of our Disorder; The Life of T. E. Lawrence*. Boston: Little, Brown and Company

Masson, J. Moussaieff. 1992. *Assault on Truth: Freud's Suppression of the Seduction Theory*. New York: HarperPerennial.

Maté, Gabor. 2008. *In the Realm of Hungry Ghosts: Close Encounters with Addiction*. Toronto: Knopf Canada.

Miller, Alice. 2008. *The Drama of the Gifted Child: The Search for the True Self*. New York: Basic Books.

Milne, A. A. 1927. *Now We Are Six*. London. E. P. Dutton.

Montagu, Ashley. 2010. *Touching: The Human Significance of Skin*. Memphis, Tenn: General Books.

Neill, A.S. 1960. *Summerhill: A Radical Approach to Child Rearing*. New York: Hart Pub. Co.

Passie, Torsten. 2012. *Healing with Entactogens: Therapist and Patient Perspectives on MDMA-assisted Group Psychotherapy*. Santa Cruz,

Calif.: Multidiscplinary Association for Psychedelic Studies (MAPS).

Perry, Bruce Duncan. 2006. *The Boy Who Was Raised as a Dog: And Other Stories from a Child Psychiatrist's Notebook: What Traumatised Children Can Teach Us About Loss, Love, and Healing.* New York: Basic Books.

Ray, Reginald. 2016. *The Awakening Body: Somatic Meditation for Discovering Our Deepest Life.* Boulder: Shambhala.

Reich, Wilhelm. 2013. *Character Analysis.* New York: Farrar, Straus and Giroux.

Smith, Huston. 2000. *Cleansing the Doors of Perception.* New York: Jeremy P. Tarcher/Putnam.

Stolaroff, Myron J. 2004. *The Secret Chief Revealed.* Sarasota, Fl.: Multidisciplinary Association for Psychedelic Studies (MAPS).

Taylor, Kylea and Jack Kornfield. 1995. *The Ethics of Caring: Honoring the Web of Life in Our Professional Healing Relationships.* Second edition. Hanford Mead.

Whitaker, Robert. 2015. *Anatomy of an Epidemic: Magic Bullets, Psychiatric Drugs, and the Astonishing Rise of Mental Illness in America.* New York: Broadway Books.

And, also...

Adamson, Sophia. 2012. *Through the Gateway of the Heart: Accounts of Experiences with MDMA and Other Empathogenic Substances.* Petaluma, Calif.: Solarium Press.

This unique and special book deserves particular mention and an affirmative shout-out. During the many years since Carl B. presented the essay that inspired us to begin the process of assembling his and all the other testimonies into this volume, we attended a gathering of likeminded souls in Lisbon where we were introduced to the second edition of the book, *Through the Gateway of the Heart* by Sophia Adamson, republished in 2012. The first edition had been published in 1985 just as MDMA, then affectionately known as Adam, was placed on Schedule 1. The book, therefore, did not have the opportunity to reach the wide audience it deserved and publication was discontinued.

We were delighted to find that the authors, Ralph Metzner, PhD, and Padma Catell, PhD, had chosen to present their clients' experiences through over fifty testimonies, prefiguring our own MO by decades. To read their accounts of the experiences and outcomes from the original iteration of MDMA's use in a therapeutic context was affirming, and our own first testimony, from Elly S., took place around that time. We feel great fraternity with both participants and authors and sincerely recommend *Through the Gateway of the Heart* to readers who might wish to seek additional firsthand evidence of the healing potential of this extraordinary medicine.

So, from across an ocean, a continent and thirty years, we collectively give a deep bow of gratitude, love and respect to their original work.

. . .

Readers who may wish to seek engagement with issues surrounding MDMA, including clinical research and efforts to remove the Schedule 1 prohibition, are respectfully directed toward the following organisations:

In the UK, The Beckley Foundation is a think-tank and NGO whose purpose is to drive evidence-based drug policy reform. http://beckleyfoundation.org.

In the US, The Multidisciplinary Association for Psychedelic Studies, (MAPS) directs funding and research endeavours that include their fierce advocacy of the healing potential of MDMA when it is respected as a medicine. www.maps.org.

Readers may also be interested to see the following information-rich video:

Treating Trauma; A Discussion with Richard Rockefeller, M.D. and Larry Brilliant, M.D.

https://www.youtube.com/watch?v=wE8jEXksn7Q

Additionally, entering the words trauma, PTSD and MDMA into a search engine will bring readers to a wide variety of presentations including articles, videos, and blogs.

Thank you.

"Of all the motions and conditions of the Soul,
Love is the only one by means of which we can
treat with the Creator
and give back something resembling
that which we have been given."

ANONYMOUS

43407379R00258

Made in the USA
Middletown, DE
23 April 2019